Advancing Breastfeeding:
Forging Partnerships
for a
Better Tomorrow

Praeclarus Press, LLC
2504 Sweetgum Lane
Amarillo, Texas 79124 USA
806-367-9950
www.PraeclarusPress.com

DISCLAIMER
The information contained in this publication is advisory only and is not intended to replace sound clinical judgment or individualized patient care. The author disclaims all warranties, whether expressed or implied, including any warranty as the quality, accuracy, safety, or suitability of this information for any particular purpose.

ISBN: 978-1-939807-44-1

Cover Design: Ken Tackett
Illustrations: Ken Tackett
Copy Editing: Chris Tackett
Acquisition & Development: Kathleen Kendall-Tackett
Layout & Design: Nelly Murariu
Operations: Scott Sherwood

Advancing Breastfeeding:
Forging Partnerships
for a
Better Tomorrow

Papers from the 9th Breastfeeding and Feminism International Conference

March 20-21, 2014

Sheraton Chapel Hill, Chapel Hill, NC

EDITORS

MIRIAM LABBOK, MD, MMS, MPH, IBCLC; FACPM, FABM, FILCA; Carolina Global Breastfeeding Institute Founding Professor and Director; Department of Maternal and Child Health, Gillings School of Global Public Health, University of North Carolina at Chapel Hill

PAIGE HALL SMITH, MSPH, PhD; Associate Professor, Public Health Education, Director Center for Women's Health and Wellness, School of Health and Human Sciences, University of North Carolina at Greensboro

Praeclarus Press, LLC

www.PraeclarusPress.com

Table of Contents

Section I   1

Forging Partnerships Across the Socioecology Framework: Global, National, State, Organizational, and Community

This volume opens with examples of how different communities have reached out to partner to advance protection, promotion, and support of breastfeeding at the global, national, state, and local levels. The first two papers explore international issues, and the next two address national issues, first in Haiti and then in the U.S. Two papers address state-level activities and we conclude with a special city-level activity prioritizing partnering.

Section II   69

Forging Partnerships with Diverse Communities to Reduce Disparities in Breastfeeding and Increase Equity in Outcomes

This section addresses the challenges of common messaging–breastfeeding—across diverse cultural and racial populations. The first paper addresses the underlying issues, while the next two address issues encountered by the African American mother, followed by two considering immigrant communities. Three papers addressing the challenges of LGBTQ parenting are followed by the special issue of breastfeeding among incarcerated women.

Section III   123
Forging Partnerships within the Health Care Community

Central to the consideration of breastfeeding and feminism is the reality of the positive health outcomes associated with breastfeeding. This chapter focuses first on issues that arise in the practice of breastfeeding support, and then on issues related to support by providers.

Section IV   215
Forging Partnerships to Increase Community Support for Women, Children, and Families

Breastfeeding is a socially and culturally based behavior; women generally need the help of others to succeed with breastfeeding. This section explores several parts of our environment that deserve attention as potential partners.

IVa. Breastfeeding in the Community: Sharing Health

IVb. Breastfeeding and Women's Lives   243

Section V   275
Partnering through Narrative: Social Media and Communications

We conclude this volume with several papers addressing the real issues in partnering and communication, even within the breastfeeding and the feminist communities. Social media and other communications media are playing an increasing role in our discourse. Here we see both the supportive and challenging aspects of narratives and media experiences as breastfeeding is becoming increasingly accepted as normative in all societies.

Foreword

The Breastfeeding and Feminism International Conference (BFIC) series was initially designed to raise the profile of breastfeeding within the women's advocacy and feminist studies' communities, and to increase recognition among breastfeeding supporters that breastfeeding promotion could receive more sociopolitical support by partnering with those concerned with women's reproductive health, rights, and justice; women's economic advancement; emerging sexual, gender, and feminist issues; and the elimination of social, economic, and health inequities.

The theme of the ninth conference, the 2014 Breastfeeding and Feminism International Conference, *Advancing Breastfeeding: Forging Partnerships for a Better Tomorrow,* reflects the reality that, while breast-feeding is of growing interest to many in the disciplines of health, sociology, and anthropology, we still have an insufficient number of partners outside of these professional interest groups. If we wish to make a difference for women and their desire to breastfeed in our current commerciophilic and technophilic society, it is vital to build synergistic partnerships in order to create a voice that will be heard by high-level policy makers. Such partnerships should enable those working on feminism and breastfeeding, and related reproductive health, to bridge gaps, explore intersectional ties, and to break down silos in order to strengthen policy and action through collaboration, mutual action, and advocacy.

Please note that the conference declares that it did not accept funding from any organization that violates the International Code of Marketing of Breast-milk Substitutes and subsequent resolutions. Despite this clear declaration, one speaker declared upon arrival that she does accept funding from a Code violator. According to the Code, if a health care provider accepts research funding, they must declare so. In this case, the speaker declared her conflict and was included in this volume. No other speaker declared any related COI.

This volume is divided into broad sections with chapters that offer several papers addressing differing aspects of the issue. Many of the speakers who contributed chapters to this volume address the theme of forging partnerships at the global, national, state, and cultural levels, and across disciplines and fields of endeavor. Concerning forging partnerships, we, as organizers, were surprised that this call received minimal traction with those in the family planning and maternal reproductive health arena. This gap merits further discussion in the context of both feminism and preventive health care, and we hope to address this in the future.

Other chapters in each section of this volume continue the conference's overriding focus on feminism and breastfeeding, disparities in service and inequity in outcomes, women's reproductive health and clinical support, community support and social media, and women's issues. Finally, we continue our attention to historical perspectives with thanks to the ongoing contributions of Dr. Jacqueline Wolf.

We hope you enjoy this volume.

Miriam Labbok, MD, MPH, IBCLC
Paige Hall Smith, PhD

Contributing Authors

Kathleen L. Anderson, MEd, CLC, is director of Community Breastfeeding at the Carolina Global Breastfeeding Institute where she implements a statewide Breastfeeding-Friendly Child Care project and coordinates a project studying breastfeeding services from day 2 to week 12 postpartum. She also facilitates a national collaborative on advancing breastfeeding in child care. Kathleen has a Master's degree in Education with focus on Early Intervention and Family Support. She is a Certified Lactation Counselor and La Leche League Leader.

Erica Hesch Anstey, PhD, is currently an ORISE fellow with the Nutrition Branch of the Centers for Disease Control and Prevention (CDC), where she works with the Infant Feeding Team on translating research into guidance. She received her PhD in public health from the University of South Florida in Tampa, where she worked on the study presented in these conference proceedings. She also has an MA in women's studies and is a certified lactation counselor (CLC). Erica has long been interested in becoming a leader in Maternal and Child Health (MCH) and was an MCH Trainee (2011-2012). She is a member of the International Affiliation of Tongue-Tie Professionals and is a member of the Editorial Review Board for the *Journal of Human Lactation*. Her research interests include breastfeeding management issues, tongue-tie, breastfeeding disparities, and family-centered care. She has worked on several studies related to breastfeeding including a community needs assessment for a university-led clinical lactation program, and her dissertation on International Board Certified Lactation Consultants' (IBCLCs') perceived professional barriers to managing early breastfeeding problems. Erica is particularly interested in bridging the disciplines of feminist studies and public health as a way to improve maternal and child health outcomes and delivery of care.

Emily Anzicek, PhD, in Communication, Wayne State University, 2007, is the Director of Introduction to Public Speaking and an instructor in the Department of Communication at Bowling Green State University in Ohio. Her current research explores the potential role of media in normalizing breastfeeding in American culture. Her doctoral dissertation explored the representations of teen sex and its consequences in four television shows that aired on the former WB television network.

Yeon Bai, PhD, RD, has many years of experience as a registered dietitian at WIC clinics, which enriched her understanding of issues and concerns important to mothers, as well as the importance of environmental support to practice breastfeeding. She employs both qualitative and quantitative methodology to explore and examine factors associated with breastfeeding rates. In her research, she uses behavioral theories to understand why mothers do or don't breastfeed in an effort to provide guidelines for effective promotion strategies. Her research extends to improve environmental support, including hospitals and workplaces. She is an Associate Professor in the Department of Health and Nutrition Sciences at Montclair State University.

Cecilia E. Barbosa, PhD, MPH, MCP, is principal cBe consulting. She received a PhD in social and behavioral health from Virginia Commonwealth University in December 2014; her dissertation was on infant feeding barriers and facilitators among low-income African American women in Richmond. She has worked for over 20 years in public health in Virginia, as an independent consultant, as Director, Division of Child and Adolescent Health, and as Director of Planning and Evaluation, Division of Maternal and Child Health, Virginia Department of Health. She received Master of Public Health and Master of City Planning degrees from the University of California at Berkeley. She serves on the Governor of Virginia's Latino Advisory Board, the Virginia Department of Health Institutional Review Board, the Mayor of Richmond's Breastfeeding Taskforce, and Virginia Public Health Association board. She is fluent in Portuguese, Spanish, and French.

Chantal Bayard graduated in social work at Université de Montréal in 1999 and for 5 years, she worked as a community organizer in two local health centers (CLSC) in Montreal. In 2008, she obtained a master's degree in sociology at Université du Québec à Montréal with her thesis entitled "Social Representations of Breastfeeding Among Pregnant Quebec Women who Want to Breastfeed." She has several years of experience as a research assistant and worked two years as a project manager in a public health non-profit organization. In 2014, she edited a collective work entitled "Promotion of Breastfeeding in Quebec: A Critical Perspective" (*Les Éditions du remue-ménage*). She is a doctoral student in sociology at University of Ottawa.

Kellie E. Carlyle, PhD, MPH, is Associate Professor and Program Director in the Department of Social and Behavioral Health in the School of Medicine and affiliate faculty in the Center for Media + Health and Institute for Women's Health at Virginia

Commonwealth University. She holds a PhD in Social and Behavioral Sciences and MPH in Health Behavior, and Health Promotion from The Ohio State University. Dr. Carlyle was named a Centennial Professor for excellence in teaching, mentoring, and community engagement in her previous position at Arizona State University and has received multiple Community Engagement grants from VCU. She publishes and teaches in the areas of health behavior theory; campaign design, implementation and evaluation; women's health; violence prevention; and sexual health promotion.

Ellen Chetwynd BSN, MPH, IBCLC, is a PhD candidate at the University of North Carolina at Chapel Hill and a lactation consultant at an out of hospital birth center. She has been a lactation consultant for fifteen years, and worked extensively in maternal and child health as a clinician and in management. The education she is receiving in epidemiologic methods allows for direct translational research from the clinical setting to the academic and scientific spheres as well as the application of implementation science in the study of and advocacy for systems of breastfeeding support. Her publications cover topics in advocacy for the profession of lactation consulting, as well as explorations of breastfeeding difficulties, breastfeeding support systems, and the biological make up of human milk. She is an adamant supporter of diverse breastfeeding populations, and has published on the intricacies of two-mother families, as well as working on several projects engaging minority populations. Her dissertation work will explore the association between breastfeeding and metabolic health in a large cohort of African American women.

Rachel M Davis, MPH, RD, grew up in Columbia, South Carolina. In 2010, she received her Bachelor's degree in Nutritional Sciences from Pennsylvania State University. She recently received her Master's in Public Health in December of 2013 from the Department of Maternal and Child Health at the University of North Carolina Chapel Hill. She is a Registered Dietitian and an International Board Certified Lactation Consultant currently employed with the Department of Health and Human Services (DHHS) in the Special Supplemental Nutrition Program for Women Infants and Children (WIC) in Monroe, North Carolina.

Joan E. Dodgson PhD, MPH, FAAN, is an Associate Professor at Arizona State University and the Executive Director of the Southwest Clinical Lactation Education Program. Her research interests include infant feeding, breastfeeding, effects of culture, perinatal nursing, community-based, qualitative methods, Asia, and nursing philosophy.

Kirsten Doehler, PhD, holds the position of Associate Professor of Statistics at Elon University where she is the Statistics Program Coordinator. She received her doctorate in Statistics at North Carolina State University in 2006. Dr. Doehler's diverse research agenda includes projects related to statistical consulting, statistics education, sports analytics, and biostatistics. Her peer-reviewed papers have appeared in social science and natural science journals, statistics education journals, and in one of the top medical statistics journals. In 2014, Dr. Doehler became a SAS Software Certified Base Programmer.

Laura E. Downey, BSN, graduated 2002 with BS in Public Health (Environmental Sciences and Engineering major; Biology minor) from UNC Chapel Hill and worked for several years on public health issues, particularly as they related to environmental quality (e.g., air pollution, water pollution, community-wide pesticide spraying). In 2009, she decided to change careers and to pursue nursing, a field in which she felt she could make more of a direct impact on people's lives. She graduated in 2010 from the Accelerated Bachelors of Science in Nursing program at UNC Chapel Hill with highest honors for her honors project entitled, "Breastfeeding Cessation: Associations with Maternal Depression and Infant Temperament in African-American Mothers." Since graduating, she has worked on the 31-bed Neurosciences unit at Duke University Hospital.

Spring-Serenity Duvall, PhD, is an Assistant Professor of Communications at the University of South Carolina, Aiken. She completed her PhD in Journalism and Mass Communication at Indiana University (2010) with a minor in Gender Studies. Her research on celebrity culture, girlhood studies, and commodity activism has appeared in *Communication, Culture, and Critique; Journal of Children and Media;* in the edited volumes *Circuits of Visibility: Gender and Transnational Media Cultures* by Radha Hegde and *Celebrity Colonialism: Fame, Representation, and Power in Colonial and Post-Colonial Cultures* by Robert Clarke; and a forthcoming article in *Feminist Media Studies*. She has presented research at annual conferences for the International Communication Association, the Political Studies Association (UK), the National Communication Association (USA), the Society for Cinema and Media Studies, and the Association of Educators in Journalism and Mass Communication (USA), where she is currently chair of the Commission on the Status of Women.

Laurel Falconi, MA, graduated in sociology from the University of Ottawa, Ontario, Canada this past year, upon completing her Honors Bachelor of Science from the University of Toronto, Ontario, Canada. Her research in the area of gender categorization and identities focused on transgender people in the workplace, specifically exploring how coworkers responded to working with a transgender woman. She coauthored an article about breastfeeding and gender roles in lesbian-parent households and is currently looking at female empowerment through sexual education. She also has experience researching social inequalities and mental health issues, particularly gambling and its impact on the individual and the workplace.

Katherine Foss, PhD, has explored media coverage of breastfeeding in advertising, magazines, reality television and entertainment television. Her work has appeared in numerous peer-reviewed journals, including *Health Communication, Disability Studies Quarterly, Women & Health,* and the *International Breastfeeding Journal.* She has previously presented her research at the 2013, 2010, and 2011 Breastfeeding & Feminism conferences. She was an invited speaker at the 2012 Great Nurse-In, a breastfeeding advocacy event held on the West Lawn of Capitol Hill in Washington, D.C. Dr. Foss is an Assistant Professor at Middle Tennessee State University, where she teaches courses in women and the media, health communication, and entertainment studies. She earned her Master's and PhD in Mass Communication from the University of Minnesota.

Bette Gebrian, BSN, MPH, PhD, a public health nurse and medical anthropologist, has lived and worked in rural Haiti for over 28 years. She is currently the Assistant Clinical Professor at the University of Connecticut, Department of Community Medicine. Bette directed the public health program for the Haitian Health Foundation (HHF) for 27 years and published extensively in areas of maternal and child health. She continues to work in health and development.

Jane Grassley, PhD, joined the Boise State University School of Nursing faculty in 2010 after teaching at Texas Woman's University where she earned her PhD in Nursing Science and a Graduate Certificate in Women's Studies in 2004. As an International Board-Certified Lactation Consultant (IBCLC), her research explores issues related to promoting breastfeeding. She is particularly interested in the cultural context in which breastfeeding support takes place. Her current research evaluates effective interventions for improving the breastfeeding support that mothers receive from nurses and from grandmothers. She is particularly interested in evaluating supportive nurse behaviors that optimize the childbirth and early breastfeeding experiences of adolescent mothers and their newborns. Her teaching of undergraduate nursing students provides many opportunities to be a breastfeeding advocate. She also holds a joint appointment with Women's Services at St. Luke's Regional Health System to collaboratively develop research projects with the Treasure Valley hospitals' lactation consultants.

Tyra Toston Gross, MPH, is a doctoral candidate at the University of Georgia (UGA) College of Public Health. Tyra is currently completing her qualitative dissertation on using the Positive Deviance approach to explore the breastfeeding experiences of African American women participating in the Georgia WIC program. She has her MPH degree from LSU Health Sciences Center and a B.S. in Nutritional Sciences from Louisiana State University. Tyra also has graduate certificates in Global Health, Nonprofit Management, and Qualitative Research from UGA. Tyra's short-term goal is to continue researching maternal and child health disparities in a postdoctoral fellowship. Her long-term career goals return to her home-state of Louisiana, which has the lowest breastfeeding rates, to live in New Orleans and work in the field of public health to address health disparities and social injustices. In her spare time, Tyra enjoys serving at her church and in her community.

Virginia Guidry PhD, MPH, is a postdoctoral fellow in the Department of Epidemiology at the University of North Carolina at Chapel Hill. She studies the impact of air pollutants on communities with a focus on environmental justice and community-based research. Her current research is examining the respiratory health effects experienced by children who attend schools near industrial livestock operations.

Yiota Kitsantas, PhD, MS, Associate Professor of Biostatistics and Epidemiology in Health Administration and Policy, focuses on the application of data mining techniques, such as classification and regression trees, and methods of categorical data analysis to investigate public health related issues in the fields of maternal and infant health and substance abuse among adolescents. She serves as a biostatistics consultant on numerous projects. Dr. Kitsantas has published several manuscripts in both statistical and epidemiological related peer-reviewed journals. She has also presented her research findings at national and international conferences.

Miriam Labbok, MD, MPH, IBCLC, is the Carolina Global Breastfeeding Institute Professor and Director in the Department of MCH at the University of North Carolina, Chapel Hill. Her previous work at Georgetown and Hopkins Universities, UNICEF and USAID on breastfeeding and family-planning global issues, and more recent work in North Carolina have been recognized with honors from her alma maters, and by LLLI, ILCA, and USAID, as well as with the 2012 Carl Taylor Lifetime Achievement Award from APHA, 2013 NC-GSKF Lifetime Achievement Award, and Award for Evidence-

Based Leadership in Breastfeeding, ILCA/JHL 2014. She has published more than 100 peer-reviewed articles, more than 40 chapters, co-edited 3 books, with 3 in preparation, dozens of monographs, and 100s of scientific presentations. Dr. Labbok is pleased to serve as the co-director of the Breastfeeding and Feminism International Conference.

Saba Masho, MD, MPH, DrPH, is Associate Professor of Family Medicine and Population Health and Obstetrics and Gynecology at Virginia Commonwealth University (VCU) with expertise in Maternal and Child Health Epidemiology. She is the director of Community Based Participatory Research at the VCU Institute of Women's Health, a Federally-designated Center of Excellence in Women's Health. Dr. Masho is a principal investigator and co-investigator of multiple federally funded research projects in the area of perinatal health, provision of comprehensive care to underserved pregnant women, and youth violence. She has authored numerous peer-reviewed manuscripts and given several national scientific presentations. Her recent article examining the association between BMI and breastfeeding was featured in the *Breastfeeding Medicine.*

Deborah McCarter-Spaulding, PhD, RN, is an Associate Professor of Nursing at Saint Anselm College and International Board Certified Lactation Consultant (IBCLC). Her current research is addressing an educational intervention provided by postpartum nurses and its effect on postpartum depression symptoms. She is also looking at the relationship between postpartum depression and breastfeeding. Her previous research work has also been related to breastfeeding, particularly breastfeeding confidence (self-efficacy). She is also interested in women's health, gender issues, and global health, particularly in interdisciplinary context.

Laurie L. Meschke, MS, PhD, is an Associate Professor in the Department of Public Health at the University of Tennessee, Knoxville. Laurie has over a decade of experience in conducting and disseminating research in the area of prenatal substance use and infant outcomes. While in Minnesota she examined statewide prenatal substance use, the diagnosis of Fetal Alcohol Syndrome, and the design and evaluation of a randomized-control, treatment-group evaluation of a substance abuse treatment program for high-risk women. Since moving to Tennessee in 2012, Laurie has initiated the examination of prenatal opioid use and its effects on infants.

Roger Mills-Koonce, PhD, is an Associate Professor in Human Development and Family Studies for the School of Health and Human Sciences at the University of North Carolina at Greensboro.

Chinelo Ogbuanu, MD, MPH, PhD, is a physician and graduate of the doctoral program in Health Services, Policy and Management at the Arnold School of Public Health, University of South Carolina. She possesses advanced skills in survey development and the analysis of complex surveys including the Pregnancy Risk Assessment Monitoring System (PRAMS), the Early Childhood Longitudinal Study-Birth Cohort (ECLS-B) and the National Survey of Children's Health (NSCH). She is currently a primary investigator on a study exploring the level of breastfeeding support major employers in Georgia offer their employees. She has authored multiple peer-reviewed publications as first author and co-authored a book chapter in *Comparative Health Systems: Global Perspectives*. She has also delivered several oral presentations at state, national, and international conferences. She is currently a Senior Maternal and Child Health Epidemiologist at the Georgia Department of Public Health. Her research interests include breastfeeding, maternal mortality, and perinatal health.

Beatrice Olubukola Ogunba, PhD, is a Nutritionist specializing in Maternal and Child Nutrition. Her area of research has been in breastfeeding and complementary feeding practices in Nigeria. She is currently working on a project with Nestle Foundation on the use of Drama for behavior change communication in appropriate breastfeeding and complementary feeding practices. She is a Senior Lecturer in the Department of Family, Nutrition and Consumer Sciences, Obafemi Awolowo University, Ile Ife Nigeria. Her PhD is in Public Health Nutrition from the University of Ibadan, Nigeria in 2007 and she has being working in the University as an academic staff from 1995 to date. Dr. Ogunba has 18 published journal articles and 5 conference proceedings. She is a member of 8 professional associations including the Nutrition Society of the U.K.

Hira Palla is a student at George Mason University, VA, pursuing a B.S. in Global Community Health, with a concentration in nutrition. She currently works as a Research Assistant at the Department of Health Administration and Policy, where her main research focus is on maternal and child health populations. Prior to this, she has interned as a Nutrition Assistant at various Women, Infant, and Children (WIC) clinics in Fairfax, VA as well as interned at the American Public Health Association. Her future career goals involve being a public health practitioner and researcher with a focus on maternal and child health disparities, health provider-level barriers in obtaining optimal maternal and child care, and epidemiologic and community-based methods.

Aunchalee Palmquist, PhD, Assistant Professor of Sociology and Anthropology at Elon University, is a medical anthropologist and International Board Certified Lactation Consultant (IBCLC). She received her PhD at the University of Hawaii-Manoa in 2006. Before arriving at Elon, she held a two-year appointment as Postdoctoral Associate and Lecturer at Yale University, Jackson Institute for Global Affairs, Global Health Initiative. She completed a postdoctoral fellowship at the National Institutes of Health-National Human Genome Research Institute, Social and Behavioral Research Branch from 2007-2009. Dr. Palmquist has conducted research on a wide range of topics, from healing systems in Palau to family communication about genetic test results in the U.S. She has worked in clinical, community-based, and interdisciplinary settings. She has done ethnographic fieldwork in Hawaii, Palau, and Thailand. Her current research addresses social inequalities in health, infant and child health, women's and gender studies, and science and technology studies.

Kathy Parry, MPH, IBCLC, LMBT, CEIM, is a social clinical research specialist at the Carolina Global Breastfeeding Institute (CGBI) in the Department of Maternal and Child Health at the Gillings School of Public Health, UNC-Chapel Hill. At CGBI, Kathy is the Director of Prenatal Breastfeeding Education and also leads communication efforts for the institute. Her work at CGBI has included the development of an adaptable Responsive Feeding curriculum for low-income countries, as well as research on women's perception of infant formula advertising. An International Board Certified Lactation Consultant (IBCLC) and Licensed Massage and Bodywork Therapist (LMBT), Kathy enjoys exploring how craniosacral therapy can support infants learning to breastfeed. She is a Certified Educator of Infant Massage and a former DONA-certified birth doula. Kathy received her massage therapy training in New Orleans, her undergraduate degree from UNC Chapel Hill, and her masters in Maternal and Child Health from the UNC Gillings School of Global Public Health. She is also a graduate of CGBI's Mary Rose Tully Training Initiative, a Pathway 2 program for aspiring IBCLCs.

Phyllis Rippeyoung, PhD, is an Associate Professor of Sociology at the University of Ottawa, having previously taught courses in research methods, statistics, social stratification, work, and gender, as an assistant professor at Acadia University. Her research has examined inequality in early childhood and gender inequality in pay, the workplace and in families. Her current research examines how infant feeding practices shape, and are shaped, by inequities of gender, class, and sexual orientation.

Katherine J. Roberts EdD, MPH, MCHES, is an Adjunct Associate Professor at the Teachers College of Columbia University, New York. Her research interests include evaluation of school health education programs and quality of life issues of cancer survivors.

Paola Romero, MPH, was born in Colombia, South America, where she majored in Sanitary and Environmental Engineering. She is currently in the senior year of her Master's degree in Public Health from the University of South Carolina. As an immigrant, Paola has personally witnessed and experienced the difficulties of starting a new life in an unknown place. She has also experienced the barriers and the discrimination associated with being a minority with a different culture and language, and the inequities and disadvantages Latino face in the US. Motivated by this situation and hoping to promote health and to prevent diseases among her community, Paola joined the community-based group called *Pasos,* which works for improving the health of Latino Community in SC. As a Community ambassador for this project, Paola and other members of the team are developing workshops related with social justice and sexual and reproductive health. Specifically, Paola and some members of her team develop breastfeeding workshops for Latino mothers in Richland and Lexington counties of SC, and expects to works in the future in more projects related to social justice for the Latino community in the USA. Paola participated on the South Carolina Hispanic/ Latino Health Coalition and in the Healthy South Carolina Healthy Initiative, and currently, she is participating with the Witness to Hunger project of the Drexel University in Philadelphia, PA.

Beverly Rossman, PhD, RN, is an Assistant Professor in the Department of Women, Children and Family Nursing at Rush University in Chicago. Her background is in pediatric and labor and delivery nursing, with a special emphasis on childbirth education, breastfeeding, and new-parent support groups. She co-founded Parent in Touch, to provide new parents, but particularly new mothers, with a safe haven to come and talk about breastfeeding problems, parenting stress, their own anxieties and whether they were interfering with their parenting behavior and/or their parent-child relationship. Dr. Rossman has a research program of three separate, but related qualitative studies which have evaluated NICU mothers' and health care providers' perceptions of the NICU-based breastfeeding peer-counselor practice. Dr. Rossman's peer counselor research has been published in peer-reviewed journals, and she has co-authored a book chapter on mother-to-mother support about the Rush Mothers' Milk Club peer counselors. Her current research is a qualitative study investigating maternal stress/anxiety and becoming a mother as part of a larger study investigating the relationship between mother's stress/anxiety and maternal role development, parenting, breastmilk and infant development in collaboration with a child psychologist. Future research projects include determining why mothers of very preterm infants who begin providing human milk (HM; milk from the infant's own mother) are unable to meet their own HM-feeding goals to continue providing HM at the time of NICU discharge.

Paige Hall Smith, PhD, is Professor of Public Health Education and Director of the Center for Women's Health and Wellness at the University of North Carolina at Greensboro. She is the founder and co-Director of the Breastfeeding and Feminism International Conference. She holds adjunct appointments in the Departments of Maternal and Child Health and in Health Behavior at the University of North Carolina at Chapel Hill. She has received federal, state, and local support for her research on breastfeeding and gender-based violence, has authored numerous articles and is the editor on a series of books based on presentations at the Breastfeeding and Feminism International Conference.

Catherine Sullivan, MPH, RD, LDN, IBCLC, is Clinical Instructor, Director of Training and Deputy Director for the Carolina Global Breastfeeding Institute in the Department of Maternal and Child Health at the Gillings School of Public Health, University of North Carolina at Chapel Hill. Her research interests include breastfeeding, lactation, and nutrition education and support services.

Hannah Tello, MEd, MA, is a community psychologist with a specialization in maternal and infant health. She holds degrees from the University of Massachusetts Lowell and Mount Holyoke College. She is a breastfeeding counselor, as well as the founding member of the Breastfeeding Working Group of the Greater Lowell Health Alliance. Her research focuses on ecological models of breastfeeding support and intervention, with a special interest in underrepresented groups including sexual minorities, women in poverty, and recent immigrants. Her current projects include the creation and implementation a model of breastfeeding-friendly campus policies through a social justice lens, as well as the development of culturally competent best-practice materials for clinicians working with breastfeeding parents who are sexual minorities and/or transgender. She is also mom to a toddler, Pax, and owns a custom nail polish business.

Kristin P. Tully, PhD, is a Postdoctoral Research Associate at the Carolina Global Breastfeeding Institute and Center for Developmental Science at the University of North Carolina at Chapel Hill. She obtained her PhD in Biological Anthropology from Durham University, United Kingdom, in 2010. Dr. Tully was a Postdoctoral Fellow through the Carolina Consortium on Human Development funded by the Eunice Kennedy Shriver National Institute of Child Health and Human Development from 2010 to 2013. Her program of research investigates health care and parenting decisions in the domains of childbirth and infancy, particularly around night-time breastfeeding.

Amber Valentine, MS, CCC-SLP, BCS-S, is a Speech-Language Pathologist and Certified Lactation Counselor at Baptist Health Lexington hospital. She is responsible for the care of adult/pediatric patients (including NICU) with dysphagia. The care regimen includes assessment/treatment of patients including infant and pediatric feeding evaluations, clinical bedside evaluations, Modified Barium Swallow studies, and FEES®. She works with infants and mothers in the NICU and pediatric setting to provide care for breast- and bottle-feeding with any infants with feeding difficulties, including prematurity, infants with down syndrome (and other syndromes), infants with cleft lip and/or palate, infants of diabetic mothers, IUGR, and other diagnoses. She also evaluates and provides assistant with IBCLCs in the outpatient setting for infants who continue to have difficulty with breastfeeding, including oral motor assessments, and referrals to other areas when needed.

Agustina Vidal is a lactation consultant, one of the original administrators of Human Milk 4 Human Babies Global Milksharing Network, and co-coordinator of World Milksharing Week. She has spent the past three years intimately getting to know many of the milksharing families they serve, and understanding their needs and desires. In a past life, before marriage and before children, she was a human rights worker in Buenos Aires, Argentina, with a very strong focus in public policy, having worked in grassroots movements, human rights organizations and government agencies." She is currently the program coordinator at The Icarus Project, a radical mental-health support network and media project by, and for, people who experience the world in ways that are often diagnosed as mental illness.

Amanda Watkins, MS, RD, IBCLC, is the Director for the Southwest Clinical Lactation Education Program, a Research Assistant, and PhD student in the ASU College of Nursing and Health Innovation. She has a Master's degree in Nutrition, is a Registered Dietitian, and a practicing IBCLC. During her 20 years working in maternal and child health, she has provided consultations and taught college-level professional lactation courses. Ms. Watkins' research interest is breastfeeding educational interventions for health care providers.

Elizabeth Wierman, MSW, is a social worker in Seattle, WA and research assistant at the University of Washington's School of Social Work. Her research interests include maternal health, social determinants of health, health disparities, and addiction. She is interested in utilizing mixed methods approaches in research that advances the wellbeing of women and disadvantaged populations. Elizabeth holds a BA degree in Sociology with a concentration in Women's Studies from Gonzaga University, and a M.S.W degree with an emphasis on Integrated Health/Mental Health from the University of Washington.

Kathryn M. Webb is a first year Master's student in Public Health at the University of Tennessee, Knoxville, where she also received her undergraduate degree in Child and Family Studies. With a strong interest in child development, Kathryn has a great deal of work and volunteer experience with children. Last spring, she interned at Knox County Health Department and worked alongside health educators to create, implement, and evaluate nutritional lessons for after-school centers in Knox County. Currently, Kathryn works under the direction of Dr. Laurie L. Meschke as a graduate research assistant exploring breastfeeding among mothers in treatment for opioid use.

Jacqueline H. Wolf, PhD, is Professor of the History of Medicine in the Department of Social Medicine at Ohio University. She specializes in the history of women's and children's health and medicine, the history of public health, and the history of biomedical ethics. Her research focuses on the history of birth and breastfeeding practices in the United States. Her articles have appeared in many venues including the *American Journal of Public Health, Women and Health, Journal of Social History, Journal of Women's History, Signs, Journal of Human Lactation, Breastfeeding Medicine* and, most recently, *The Milbank Quarterly*, which ran as a featured article in the December 2013 issue the article she co-authored with her brother about end-of-life care in the United States using their mother's death from lung cancer in 2010 as a case study. She is also the author of two books, *Don't Kill Your Baby: Public Health and the Decline of Breastfeeding in the 19th and 20th Centuries* (Ohio State University Press, 2001) and *Deliver Me from Pain: Anesthesia and Birth in America* (Johns Hopkins University Press, 2009). She is currently writing a book-length social history of cesarean section in the United States, to be published by Johns Hopkins University Press in 2017. Her research on cesarean section is supported by a three-year

National Institutes of Health Scholarly Works in Medicine and Health grant.

Susan Young, PhD, recently retired from the University of Exeter, UK, where she taught and researched in the fields of childhood studies, early childhood education, and music education. She trained originally as a pianist, and worked as a school teacher, before gaining her first university position more than 20 years ago. She has a PhD from the University of Surrey, which focuses on spontaneous music play in early childhood. Determined to lead an active retirement, she enrolled on a further post-graduate research degree in anthropology at the University of Bristol. The focus of this degree on infant feeding among Somali women in the city brings together many long-standing interests; in infancy, in the refugee and recently arrived Muslim communities in the UK, and in breastfeeding; all of which she has prior experience through research projects and teaching carried out in her university position.

Seeking Synergy to Enhance Impact And Action

Miriam H. Labbok

The theme of this book encourages us to consider whether or not we might be able to find partners in our quest to support women in their breastfeeding intentions. Perhaps we need to start close to breastfeeding's physiology and consider if we might partner with those who support maternal health, recognizing the need for consideration of both mother and child, as well as healthy birth and child spacing. We also must consider other associated preventive interventions, such as prevention of high BMI and decreasing health disparities.

Our understanding of why breastfeeding is important can mediate how we act and with whom we choose to partner. Perhaps the closest linkage is between breastfeeding and birth activities. The hospital practices that disrupt women's birth experiences, and on those that disrupt breastfeeding and exclusive breastfeeding success, are closely aligned. Improving those practices begins with respecting the health and resilience of both the mother and the newborn. There is no question that birth-related practices impact breastfeeding initiation and success. Listening to Mothers II: Second National U.S. Survey of Women's Childbearing Experiences (http://www.childbirthconnection.org/pdfs/LTMII_report.pdf) found that, despite the primarily healthy population in the U.S., the majority of mothers experienced invasive procedures, such as continuous fetal monitoring, multiple vaginal exams, IV drip, epidural or spinal analgesia, and urinary catheterization. Half of the mothers experienced induction, and about a third experienced abdominal delivery. To summarize, the vast majority of women had significant disruption of the normal physiological flow from, at, or before the onset of labor through the initiation and establishment of successful breastfeeding.

Therefore, we should be partnering in the development of Mother/Baby-Friendly practices, and woman-centered and centering care. One proven intervention to support women in breastfeeding is the Baby-Friendly Hospital Initiative, with its Ten Steps to Successful Breastfeeding. Both CIMS and IMBCO have supported the implementation of Ten Steps that enhance the safety of birthing practices. This is a partnering opportunity that serves health, supports maternal informed decisions, and improved breastfeeding.

Another area where partnership seems obvious is the possibility of program and policy synergies between breastfeeding and family planning. The physiological impact of breastfeeding on fertility is a natural complement to the desire for adequate birth spacing for health of the mother and child. However, few in the family planning community have expanded their view beyond contraceptive technologies to include recognition of the ability of women to understand their own fertility and reliably switch to another method when, for example, the Lactational Amenorrhea Method no longer applies. Much work remains to create a solid and universal partnership between these two extremely complementary areas of interest.

There are certainly partnerships to build with labor unions and employers, as more and more families depend on two incomes. Where maternity and family leave are limited, such as in the U.S., it is vital to seek partnerships with those who help select workplace benefits. Co-located childcare, paid leave, and job security both attract young employable families, but also help retain workers.

The breastfeeding community must also be more proactive in creating partnerships with global MCH policies and programs. Logically, the breastfeeding community should look first to those activities designed to improve nutrition and those that reach mothers and children in their early days, months, and years of life. Those interested in the new mother-newborn initiatives, the first 1000 days, immunization campaigns, social development goals, or even human rights and many other policy and action areas are logical and essential partners to pursue for the further support of mothers to decide to breastfeed optimally and to succeed with their decisions.

Finally, any organization that purports to support a better life should be open to partnering with breastfeeding organizations. Churches and other faith-based organizations, gender-supportive groups, sororities and fraternities, international groups developed to advance social well-being (such as Rotary), and local groups working to improve life and health are reasonable allies and partners.

We who work to support breastfeeding must do more to reach out and create these partnerships, and breakdown the silos that keep us apart. Each of us can, and must, act to create change through creating partnerships to go forward together.

Forging Partnerships across the Socioecology Framework: Global, National, State, Organizational, and Community

The World Alliance for Breastfeeding Action: A Global Partnership

Miriam Labbok, MD, MPH, IBCLC

O ne of the longest standing global alliances in support of breastfeeding is the World Alliance for Breastfeeding Action (WABA), founded February 14, 1991. Its founding was preceded by the development of the International Baby Food Action Network (IBFAN), dedicated primarily to support for the Code of Marketing, La Leche League International (LLLI), dedicated to mother-to-mother support, International Lactation Consultant Association (ILCA), the global association of Lactation Consultants, and Wellstart, International, a global training program, all of which became Core Partners with WABA. Later, the Academy of Breastfeeding Medicine also became a Core Partner, dedicated to physician education. Other organizations supportive of the development of WABA include UNICEF as the major sponsor, American Public Health Association, Consumers Unions (IOCU), and World Council of Churches (WCC).

WABA is a global network of individuals and organizations concerned with protecting, promoting, and supporting breastfeeding worldwide. Its actions are based on the 1990 *Innocenti Declaration*, and later, the *Ten Links for Nurturing the Future, Global Strategy for Infant and Young Child Feeding,* and *Innocenti + 15.* WABA is in consultative status with UNICEF and an NGO in Special Consultative Status with the Economic and Social Council of the United Nations (ECOSOC).

WABA's Vision is: A world where breastfeeding is the cultural norm, where mothers and families are enabled to feed and care optimally for their infants and young children, thus contributing to a just and healthy society.

Its Mission is: To protect, promote and support breastfeeding worldwide in the framework of the *Innocenti Declarations* (1990 and 2005) and the *Global Strategy for Infant and Young Child Feeding* through networking, and facilitating collaborative efforts in social advocacy, information dissemination, and capacity building.

WABA is constantly working towards its goal, which is to foster a strong and cohesive breastfeeding movement, which will act on the various international instruments to create an enabling environment for mothers, thus contributing to increasing optimal breastfeeding and infant and young child feeding practices.

To better understand WABA's special role, it is helpful to know the operational targets of the 1990 *Innocenti Declaration on the Protection, Promotion and Support of Breastfeeding*. This document, signed by more than 30 nations, called for all nations to:

1. Appoint a national breastfeeding coordinator of appropriate authority and establish a multi-sectoral national breastfeeding committee.

2. Ensure that every facility providing maternity services fully practices all *Ten Steps to Successful Breastfeeding.*

3. Give effect to the principles and aim of the International Code of Marketing of Breast-Milk Substitutes and subsequent relevant Health Assembly resolutions in their entirety.

4. Enact imaginative legislation protecting the breastfeeding rights of working women and establish means for its enforcement.

5. Later, when the *Global Strategy for Infant and Young Child Feeding* added five additional operational targets, WABA adopted them as well, calling for every nation to:

6. Create Comprehensive policy on infant and young child feeding.

7. Support the goal of Exclusive breastfeeding for six months.

8. And the goal of Timely, adequate, safe and appropriate complementary feeding with continued breastfeeding.

9. Provide guidance on feeding infants and young children in exceptionally difficult circumstances.

10. Consider what new legislation or other suitable measures may be required.

The Alliance also recognized the *Ten Links for Nurturing the Future*, in the box, below.

---

1. HUMAN RIGHTS AND RESPONSIBILITIES
2. FOOD SECURITY through support of breastfeeding
3. WOMEN'S EMPOWERMENT through innovative social support systems
4. COMMUNITY PARTICIPATION encouraging development of community support groups and involvement of the entire community
5. BABY-FRIENDLY CULTURES including the *Ten Steps to Successful Breastfeeding* in the health care system and expanding the "baby-friendly" concept
6. INTEGRITY emphasizing avoidance of conflict of interest
7. INTERNATIONAL Code of Marketing of Breastmilk Substitutes and subsequent relevant World Health Assembly Resolutions
8. CAPACITY BUILDING
9. ADVOCACY for the implementation of the promotion, protection, and support of breastfeeding
10. SOCIAL MOBILIZATION

Exclusive Breastfeeding: the Gold Standard

SAFE, SOUND, SUSTAINABLE

THE GOLDEN BOW

is a symbol for the "Gold Standard", that is the ideal, of exclusive and continued breastfeeding.

One loop represents the mother and the other represents the child. The knot symbolises the father, family and society which support them. One of the ends is for timely complementary food after six months, the other is for the use of family planning to space births three to five years apart.

The Golden Bow is a joint outreach initiative of UNICEF and WABA. Wear it proudly and tell others if its many meanings.

For more information, visit <http://www.unicef.org/ programme/breastfeeding/bow.htm> and <www.waba.org.my /forum2/goldenbow.html>.

WABA   unicef

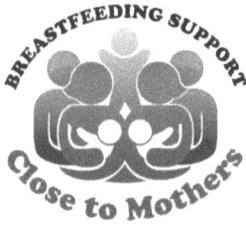

WABA is perhaps best known around the globe for World Breastfeeding Week http:// worldbreastfeedingweek.org/. This year (2014), World Breastfeeding Week will be celebrated for its 23rd year. More than 170 countries participate and the annual themes have been endorsed by all the Core Partners, as well as by WHO and UNICEF and thousands of other organizations and individuals. The purpose of this event is to unite breastfeeding advocates, governments, and agencies in a people's event with a diversity of activities and actors. Examples of the themes include the 2004 theme supporting the Golden Bow as the global symbol of exclusive breastfeeding as the Gold Standard, and 2014 celebrated peer and mother-to-mother support activities.

To learn much more about this global alliance on its webpage: http://www. waba.org.my/index.htm. Join in the celebration of World Breastfeeding Week every year, and all year long.

Conceptualizing a Mother-Baby-Breastfeeding Friendly Community: A Global Perspective

Paige Hall Smith

Overview

At the 2012 World Alliance for Breastfeeding Action Global Partners Meeting in New Delhi participants discussed the importance of identifying the key components of a breastfeeding friendly community. We have identified key "steps" to a baby-friendly hospital, and also key components of breastfeeding support at the workplace (World Health Organization, 1989). While these are critically important, a breastfeeding-friendly community would not only include, but go beyond workplace and health care support to include other structures, institutions, norms, and forces that affect women's infant feeding decisions and practices. Envisioning an ideal breastfeeding-friendly community allows us to explore possibilities, and consider what it will really take to help us achieve a community where all women are able to breastfeed and all babies have access to human milk. Identifying the key components of such a community can be challenging since communities around the world differ significantly by level of development, geography, culture, religion, resources, gender roles, women's status, labor markets, and work forces. The goal of this study was to obtain ideas from breastfeeding experts around the world about what they believe constitutes a breastfeeding-friendly community in order to develop a robust conceptualization of such a community that has global relevance.

Method

We used Delphi Methodology, an approach that gathers the opinion of experts who are not meeting face-to-face using multiple "rounds" of data collection (Stone & Busby, 1996). The second and any subsequent rounds of data collection are based on the results of the previous rounds. This study was conducted with the support of the World Alliance for Breastfeeding Action and the sample for this study were individuals affiliated with WABA as a member of the steering committee, advisory group, working group, or task force. We invited 83 such affiliated people to respond to an online questionnaire comprised primarily of open-ended questions. The sample for round two was this same group of experts plus other experts recommended by two affiliates.

Altogether, 23 people from 18 different countries participated in Study A, and 35 people from 20 countries participated in Study B. Six of the 7 major continents of the globe were represented: Asia (6), Africa (6), Europe (7), Oceana/Australia (2), North America (7), and South America (4) [Study B data].

Study A: Method and Results

For Study A, experts were given the following scenario: "Imagine that you are part of a global breastfeeding delegation that is visiting communities around the world to identify the most breastfeeding-mother-baby friendly community on the globe! You visit many different places and finally you go to one place and you know THIS IS THE ONE! THIS IS THE MOST BREASTFEEDING/MOTHER/BABY- FRIENDLY COMMUNITY IN THE WORLD!" Respondents were then given a series of questions to identify the factors across the social ecology that were at work in this community to protect, promote, and support breastfeeding. The author, and four graduate students, reviewed the qualitative data. We organized the responses into different categories and themes, and through a process of reflection and revision, we summarized the data into eight key community-level goals that are important to the development of a breastfeeding-friendly community where all women are able to breastfeed and all babies have access to human milk. We also identified objectives and strategies that might be necessary to the achievement of the goals.

Study B: Methods and Results

The questionnaire for Study Two was a quantitative instrument that asked the experts to reflect on the results derived from Study A. Specifically, respondents were asked to identify a specific community they knew well and to identify how important the eight goals and their associated objectives and strategies would be for advancing that community as one where all women are able to breastfeed and all babies have access to human milk. We also asked respondents to identify whether each item might be harmful to their community and to provide commentary. Table 1 summarizes characteristics of the specific communities considered by the respondents in Study B.

Table 1
Characteristics of Communities Visualized by Respondents

Descriptor of the Community	Response Distribution (N)		
	Generally True/Yes	Generally false/No	Not sure
Most babies are born in a hospital.	29	6	--
Over 30% of babies are born by Cesarean Section.	10	17	8
Those with low income breastfeed more than those with higher income.	11	21	2
Those with lower educational levels breastfeed more than those with higher educational levels.	10	21	3
Those who do *not* work for pay or gain breastfeed more than those who do work for pay or gain.	17	11	7
There is notable variation in breastfeeding based on cultural, racial, or ethnic background.	22	6	6
Most women work for pay or gain outside the home.	25	7	3
Boys and girls have equal access and opportunity for primary school education.	31	3	1
Boys and girls have equal access and opportunity for secondary school education.	29	5	1
Young men and women have equal access to higher education.	26	7	2
Economic, political, and social status and opportunity between men women is important in this community (1).	25	7	3
Men and women practice traditional gender roles (2)(3).	28	7	0
Women achieve high social standing primarily though being a mother (as opposed to achieving it through paid labor).	2	24	(Both) 6

1. "Generally true" combines responses: "critically important," "very important," and "somewhat important." "Generally false" combines: "not very important," and "not important at all."

2. *"Generally true" combines: "to a large extent," and "to some extent." "Generally false" consists of: "not much at all." Text responses to "other" were reviewed and then classified.*

3. Traditional gender roles were defined as men participating in the world of work and women participating as mothers, caregivers, and homemakers.

4. Excludes 3 who selected "other" as a response option.

Results from Study B indicated that most respondents, across all countries, agreed that these eight goals, and the associated objectives, are important to achieving a breastfeeding friendly community. Table 2 summarizes the eight goals and objectives; we made some revisions to the original conceptualization based on the commentaries provided by the respondents in Study B (these changes are noted in the table).

Discussion

The results of this study suggest that a "breastfeeding transition" has occurred, or is underway, in about two-thirds of the communities: this transition occurs when breastfeeding shifts from being more prolonged by women with lower, rather than higher, education to the reverse. After the transition, breastfeeding is more prolonged by women with higher, than lower, education, and income (Grummer-Strawn, 1996; Perez-Escamilla, 2003). This transition seems to follow from the confluence of several factors: increasing proportions of women employed in ways that separate them from their infants, poor workplace support for breastfeeding women, successful breastfeeding promotion efforts, and improved health care support for breastfeeding. The confluence of these factors makes breastfeeding desirable, but difficult, for many working women. Women who have more control over their work space and schedule, personal circumstances, and resources are able to breastfeed longer, and more exclusively, than their counter parts who have less control and fewer resources (Smith, 2012, 2013). Although not a condition exclusive to the far side of breastfeeding transition, there are also notable differences in breastfeeding rates by culture, and race/ethnicity. These differences may follow from the disparities by education, income, and employment.

The eight community-level goals identified in this study reflect the complex interactions between infant feeding practices and women's education, income, and employment patterns. Although each goal is individually important, each one provides only a partial solution. In some cases, the objectives needed to achieve one goal may be also help to achieve a different goal. However, there are times when the objectives that might help achieve one goal are in conflict with those used to achieve a different one. Indeed, it is also the case that the goals themselves may be in conflict at times. Hence, there are both synergies as well as tensions imbedded in the goals, objectives, and strategies. These embedded tensions make the achievement of a breastfeeding-friendly community challenging.

For example, there is widespread agreement that a breastfeeding friendly community is one that makes it possible for mothers and babies to be together (Goal 1). However, there is also widespread agreement that we also need to make it possible for mothers to success-fully integrate their maternal and occupational roles (Goal 4), and that we need to advance women's status and gender equity (Goal 5). There are, however, real tensions that exist between these three goals. It is extremely challenging in most societies to keep mothers and babies together while still ensuring that women are able to integrate their maternal and occupational roles, and advance gender equity. The biological necessity for mothers and babies to be together is one that is difficult for most and impossible for many, given the structures and policies affecting how we work, give care, and live today.

Communities around the world, including those represented by the participants in this study, vary tremendously in terms of breastfeeding rates, social/governmental support for breastfeeding, WHO Code enforcement, economic development, health sector infrastructure and care models, and women's status. Consequently, the goals, objectives, and strategies that communities use to might vary tremendously. Countries and communities have focused much attention on three of the eight goals outlined in this framework: advancing the capacity of health/medical sector to promote and support breastfeeding, ensuring the babies have access to human milk, and increasing community support for breastfeeding as the social norm. Secondarily, attention has been given to advancing strategies that enable mothers and babies to stay together, and helping women successfully integrate their maternal and occupational role. In many countries, maternity leave is a key strategy that enables women to integrate their multiple roles (Goal 4). This strategy also helps to keep mothers and babies together (Goal 1). In other countries, such as the United States, the creation of workplace lactation rooms is the key strategy we have used to help women integrate their roles. This strategy, however, does not advance the goal of keeping mothers and babies together. Going forward, more attention may need to be given to implementing strategies that focus on the goals of helping all women integrate breastfeeding, not just pumping, with paid labor (Goal 4), of ensuring good maternal breastfeeding quality of life (Goal 3), advancing women's status and gender equity (Goal 5), and reducing health and social inequities by race/ethnicity and income (Goal 8). Full implementation of the maternity protection practices recommended by the International Labor Organization (2012) would be a good strategy for helping to achieve these goals.

Table 2

Breastfeeding-Friendly Community: Goal and Objectives

Goals (# rated "critically or very important")	Objectives	# rated "critically or very important"
1. Enable mothers and babies to stay together. (35/35)	Workspaces are child and breastfeeding friendly.	33/35
	Health care providers and institutions engage in mother/baby/breastfeeding-friendly health care practices though the continuum of care (prenatal, pregnancy, birth, postpartum).	33/35
	Public breastfeeding is acceptable in all places.	28/35
2. Ensure that babies have access to human milk. [revised from: Increase the ability of mothers and others to provide human milk to babies.] (32/35)	Mothers are able to provide their own milk to their babies. [added to list of strategies based on comments from study participants.]	NA
	Donor human milk is available in the community. [revised from: Human milk is readily available in the community.]	24/34
	Adopt local polices to implement the principles set forth in the International Code of Marketing of Breastmilk Substitutes. [Revised from: The International Code of Marketing of Breast-milk Substitutes is enforced.]	33/34
	Formula is less available in the community. [Recommend deleting from objectives. Not highly endorsed, and as least one rated this as harmful.]	19/35
3. Ensure good maternal breast-feeding quality of life. (31/34)	Mothers are able to breastfeed freely and on demand.	33/34
	Breastfeeding mothers are happy breastfeeding.	33/34
	Breastfeeding mothers are proud to breastfeed.	29/34
	Breastfeeding mothers are safe from physical, psychological, and emotional harm.	30/34
	Mothers are recognized in the community as the experts of infant feeding.	27/33
	Mothers have authority over their infant feeding decisions and practices.	29/34

Goals (# rated "critically or very important")	Objectives	# rated "critically or very important"
	Mothers have support and knowledge they need to make decisions that are best for them.	34/34
	Mothers have support and knowledge they need to actualize those decisions.	34/34
4. Improve women's ability to success-fully integrate their mothering and occupational roles. (34/34)	Breastfeeding practices are flexible. By flexible, we mean that both the breastfeeding and the broader community validate different breastfeeding styles and patterns that might include feeding at the breast, pumping, and mixing breastfeeding with formula.	21/33
	Work is flexible, in that mothers have the ability to manage work. Location, time, and space.	34/34
	Mothers have access to babies while at work	32/34
	Society values mothering.	33/34
	Society values breastfeeding.	34/34
	Society values women's productive labor (paid and unpaid, formal and informal).	27/34
	Social norms support "working mothers."	25/34
	Society values children.	32/34
	Society values caregiving work.	30/34
	Women's choices about motherhood and breast-feeding do not lead to employment, discrimination, or loss of economic status.	32/34
	Mothers are healthy.	27/34
	Family and partners (fathers) support working mothers.	28/33
5. Advance women's status and gender equity. (23/34)	Gender-role norms support and value women's productive role and maternal role.	29/34
	Gender-role norms support and value paternal caregiving.	26/34
	Gender-role norms support and value paternal domestic (household) labor.	26/34

Goals (# rated "critically or very important")	Objectives	# rated "critically or very important"
	Women's bodies and breasts are not sexualized or objectified.	28/33
	Breastfeeding is recognized as a marker of women's status alongside other indicators (such as employment, education, and voting).	27/34
6. Advance the capacity of health/ medical sector to promote and support breast-feeding. (32/34)	Health care institutions practice the "10 steps."	33/34
	Health care providers and institutions engage in mother/baby/ breastfeeding-friendly health care practices though the continuum of care (prenatal, pregnancy, birth, and postpartum).	33/34
	Health care providers knowledgeable about breast-feeding- supportive practices and management of breastfeeding problems.	33/34
	Women have financial, geographic, and cultural access to quality medical/health care.	26/34
7. Increase community support for breastfeeding as the social norm. (32/34)	Traditional religious and secular leadership is supportive of breastfeeding.	22/34
	Infant feeding surveillance data is collected and used.	28/34
	Linkages between health care and various community settings are established.	27/34
	All members of the community are educated about breastfeeding.	31/34
	Women are safe and welcome to breastfeed in public spaces.	28/34
	Secular leadership is supportive of breastfeeding.	24/34
8. Reduce health and social inequities. (27/34)	All women are well nourished and healthy.	24/34
	Credible and culturally relevant breastfeeding education and support is available to minority and marginalized populations.	30/34
	Breastfeeding promotion and practice is sensitive to cultural beliefs.	30/34

References

Grummer-Strawn, L. M. (1996). The effect of changes in population characteristics on breastfeeding trends in fifteen developing countries.*International Journal of Epidemiology, 25*(1), 94-102.

Perez-Escamilla, R. (2003). Breastfeeding and the nutritional transition in the Latin American and Caribbean Region: A success story? *Cad. Saude Publica, 19* (supplement 1).

Smith, P. H. (2013). Breastfeeding and gender inequality. *Journal of Women, Politics, and Policy, 34*, 371-383.

Smith, P. H. (2012). Breastfeeding promotion through gender equity: A theoretical perspective for public health practice. In. Smith, P.H., Hausman, B.L., & Labbok, M (Eds.). *Beyond health, beyond choice: Breastfeeding constraints and realities* (pp. 33-52). New Brunswick, NJ: Rutgers University Press.

Stone Fish, L., & Busby, D. M. (1996). The Delphi method. In D. H. Sprenkle & S. M. Moon (Eds.), *Research methods in family therapy* (pp. 469–482). New York: Guilford.

World Health Organization. (1989). *Protecting, promoting, supporting breastfeeding: The special role of maternity care services. A joint WHO-UNICEF statement.* Geneva: World Health Organization.

CHAPTER 3

Environmental Impacts of Infant Feeding Choices: A Call for Collaborations

Virginia T. Guidry

Introduction

Infant feeding choices have long-term impacts on babies and their environments, yet there is limited documentation on these impacts. The 2011 *Surgeon General's Call to Action to Support Breastfeeding* includes only one paragraph on environmental impacts, and within that, only one quantitative citation (U.S. Department of Health and Human Services, 2011). A better understanding of the environmental impacts of infant-feeding choices would assist individual decisions, inform policies, and provide guidance for mitigating these impacts.

Considerations for the environmental impacts of feeding choices have been discussed in the popular media, although quantitation is typically limited. Typical considerations for impacts from infant-formula production include the generation of a dairy or soy base, packaging, shipping, bottles and nipples, energy for warming, and water/energy to clean equipment (Chait, 2009; Ecofriendly Food, 2010). Although breastfeeding doesn't require the same inputs as industrial infant-formula production, breastfeeding mothers may need to increase their caloric intake by 450 to 500 kilocalories per day (American Academy of Pediatrics, 2012). If pumping, they need a breast pump (manual or electric), energy for refrigeration or freezing, bottles/nipples, and water and energy to clean equipment.

Additionally, impacts on fertility have important environmental consequences. When infant formula is the primary source of infant nutrition, there is an earlier return of menstruation on average than with breastfeeding (Sundhagen, 2009). This can result in shorter child spacing, and possibly more children, as well as more supplies needed to manage menstruation.

Lifecycle Assessment for Infant Formula Production

Leading the effort to quantify environmental impacts of infant-feeding choices, Tinling (2011) conducted a partial lifecycle assessment (LCA) to quantify greenhouse gas emissions from infant formula production. The process of conducting an LCA typically includes attempts to quantify material extraction, manufacturing production, transportation, utilization/reuse, and disposal or recycling. Tinling (2011) focused on infant formula with a cow's milk base, and used available data from 2005.

The following steps were considered in this LCA, as summarized in Figure 1:

1. Production of cow's milk at dairy facilities,

2. Processing of pooled cow's milk at dairy plants,

3. Formula production at factories,

4. Consumer preparation of infant formula,

5. Storage of formula,

6. Transportation between production phases and to consumers, and

7. Municipal solid waste disposal.

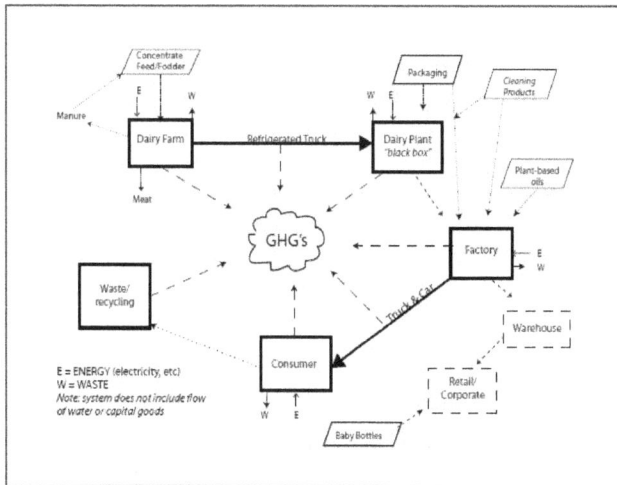

Figure 1. Lifecycle production system of powdered cows-milk-based infant formula meta-product. Source: Tinling (2011). Reproduced with permission.

Tinling found that 14.7 kilograms of carbon dioxide equivalents (CO_2-eq) are emitted per kilogram of infant formula consumed. This sums to over 2.6 million tons of CO_2-eq for total U.S. production of formula. Offsetting these emissions would cost about $8 per infant per year of consumption (Tinling, 2011).

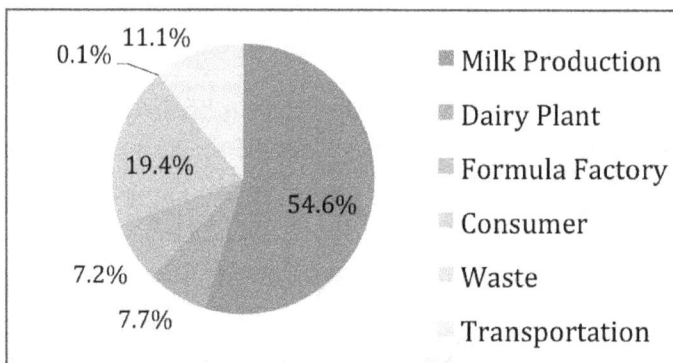

Figure 2. Relative contribution by phase to total lifecycle CO2-eq. Source: Tinling (2011). Reproduced with permission.

Relative contributions to greenhouse gas emissions from this LCA are summarized in Figure 2. The milk-production phase generates the majority (54.6%) of greenhouse gases. Consumer activities, including water heating, dishwasher use, refrigeration, and production of plastics, account for 19.4% of greenhouse gases produced. Within the transportation sector, the majority of greenhouse gases (83%) are produced during transportation from factories to retail locations (Tinling, 2011).

Toxins in Breastmilk

The ability to measure contaminants in breastmilk demonstrates that chemicals in our environment are incorporated into our bodies, and in turn, we can transfer them to our offspring during pregnancy and lactation. Many of the chemicals detected in breastmilk are lipophilic, and thus, they are stored in body fat and mobilized during lactation (Anderson & Wolff, 2000). Persistent organic pollutants, such as polychlorinated biphenyls (PCBs), dioxins, organochlorine pesticides, and polybrominated diphenyl ethers (PBDEs) are of significant concern in breastmilk because they are ubiquitous and persist in the environment, rather than breaking down over time (Anderson & Wolff, 2000; Nickerson, 2006). Heavy metals, such as lead and mercury, have known neurotoxicity, although the pharmacokinetics of these chemicals in the body, and thus their transfer to breastmilk, is poorly understood (Anderson & Wolff, 2000; American Academy of Pediatrics, 2001).

Although chemicals can be detected in breastmilk, the potential harm from these exposures is less clear. Exposures from breastmilk are often lower than those from other infant exposures routes, such as inhalation or ingestion from hand-to-mouth behavior. One study found that infant exposures to inhaled volatile organic chemicals (VOCs) were 25 to 135 times higher than exposures to VOCs from breastmilk (Kim, Halden, & Buckley, 2007). Women may terminate breastfeeding early if told that their breastmilk contains toxins (Geraghty, Khoury, Morrow, & Lamphear, 2008), although having information about these risks may mitigate their response to these concerns (Brody, Morello-Frosch, Brown, & Rudel, 2009). The National Resources Defense Council "Healthy Milk, Healthy Baby" report is a good resource for putting these results in context. It explains sources of exposure, summarizes the benefits of breastfeeding, gives suggestions for moms, and calls for breastmilk monitoring (Solomon, Weiss, Owen, & Citron, 2005).

Most importantly, at typical exposure levels, the benefits of breast-feeding such as nutrition, immune support, and mother-child bonding, far outweigh the potential impacts from chemical exposures (Anderson & Wolff, 2000). Rather, the ability to detect environmental chemicals in breastmilk should serve as a reminder that we need to minimize pollutants in the environment to protect all populations, but especially mothers and babies experiencing vulnerable developmental periods.

Call for Collaborations

Typically, breastfeeding advocacy highlights the health benefits of breastfeeding, while environmental benefits are overlooked. Established environmental and breastfeeding-advocacy groups should combine efforts to maximize both types of benefits. Some collaborations have been previously initiated, such as the call for endorsement of "Working Together for a Toxic Free Future" by the World Alliance for Breastfeeding Action (WABA) and the International Persistent Organic Pollutant Elimination Network (IPEN) (2003), but further collaborations are needed.

There is growing public interest in understanding the environmental impacts of personal choices and public-policy decisions. We know that promoting more healthful environments will also reduce chemical exposures in breastmilk. Breastfeeding experts should collaborate with environmental scientists to quantify the environmental benefits of breastfeeding compared to infant formula, and provide clear support for one more reason that breastfeeding is the best choice for infant feeding.

References

American Academy of Pediatrics. (2012). Policy statement: Breastfeeding and the use of human milk. *Pediatrics, 129*(3), e827–e841.

Anderson, H. A., & Wolff, M. S. (2000). Environmental contaminants in human milk. *Journal of Exposure Science and Environmental Epidemiology, 10,*

American Academy of Pediatrics Committee on Drugs. (2001). The transfer of drugs and other chemicals into human milk. *Pediatrics, 108*(3), 776-789.

Brody, J. G., Morello-Frosch, R., Brown, P., & Rudel, R. A. (2009). Reporting individual results for environmental chemicals in breastmilk in a context that supports breastfeeding. *Breastfeeding Medicine, 4*(2), 121.

Chait, J. (2009, Aug 11). 6 green reasons why breastfeeding is the best feeding. *Mother Nature Network*. Retrieved from http://www.mnn.com/family/family-activities/stories/6-green-reasons-why-breastfeeding-is-the-best-feeding

Ecofriendly Food. (2010). Why breastfeeding is the best choice for the environment. *Ecofriendly Food*. Retrieved from http://www.ecofriendlyfood.org.au/breastfeeding_and_the_environment

Geraghty, S. R., Khoury, J. C., Morrow, A. L., & Lamphear, B. P. (2008). Reporting individual test results of environmental chemicals in breastmilk: Potential for premature weaning. *Breastfeeding Medicine, 3*(4), 207-13.

Kim, S. R., Halden, R. U., & Buckley, T. J. (2007). Volatile organic compounds in human milk: methods and measurements. *Environmental Science and Technology, 41*(5), 1662-7.

Nickerson, K. (2006). Environmental contaminants in breast milk. *Journal of Midwifery & Women's Health, 51*(1), 26-34.

Solomon, G., Weiss, P., Owen, B., & Citron, A. (2005). Healthy milk, healthy baby: Chemical pollution and mother's milk. *Natural Resources Defense Council*. Retrieved from http://www.nrdc.org/breastmilk/

Sundhagen, R. (2009). Breastfeeding and child spacing. In H. **Selin (Ed.),** *Childbirth across cultures* (pp. 23-32). Springer: Netherlands.

Tinling, M. (2011). *Lifecycle assessment of greenhouse gas emissions of infant formula*. Unpublished thesis.

U.S. Department of Health and Human Services. (2011). *The Surgeon General's Call to Action to Support Breastfeeding*. Washington, DC: U.S. Department of Health and Human Services, Office of the Surgeon General.

World Alliance for Breastfeeding Action (WABA) & International Persistent Organic Pollutant Elimination Network (IPEN). (2003). *Working together for a toxic-free future*. Retrieved from http://www.waba.org.my/pdf/JointStatement.pdf *statement*. Geneva: World Health Organization.

Section Ib

National-Level Partnerships

CHAPTER 4

Ten Years of National and International Partnerships: A Haitian Perspective

Bette Gebrian and Kathy English

Though almost all Haitian women breastfeed their babies, the way they do so (initiation, continuation, introduction of foods, traditional purgative use, and weaning strategies) prevented children from receiving the maximum benefits that they so desperately needed. Since 1993, the Haitian Health Foundation (HHF) has worked together with mothers, grandmothers, traditional healers, nurses, community health workers, and international medical and nursing experts to build on the positive, and modify less-than-optimal behaviors.

Partnerships for family health began, as they should, with the families in the rural villages where we worked to provide basic prenatal and postpartum care. Through close relationships, we learned the traditional practices that were helpful, harmless, and some that were dangerous. Using a purgative for a newborn made of castor oil, nutmeg, and other unsavory items has been a tradition carried on by grandmothers to "clean out" the meconium stool even before breastfeeding.

As we came to understand the life ways of Haitian mothers, their mothers, healers and elders, we developed educational strategies to applaud positive practices, and addressing the most harmful ones, including cutting the umbilical cord with a non-sterile knife, or piece of glass, causing death from neonatal tetanus.

A particularly helpful collaboration, early on, was with the program at Georgetown University Institute of Reproductive Health. The Public Health Director received training in breastfeeding and the Lactation Amenorrhea Method (LAM), and brought that training back to the nurses in the HHF. Practical knowledge was key to addressing the concerns of women, and blending some traditional practices with Western knowledge. The understanding that expressed breastmilk was viable in ambient temperatures for a number of hours was an important fact permitting mothers to breastfeed exclusively and still tend to their work. Another fact particularly important for Haitian mothers, who are often malnourished themselves, is the 3-month growth spurt that temporarily outpaces milk production. Mothers said that they were poor and hungry, and that their babies' crying was an indicator that they could not feed adequately. Traditionally, this is the point when mothers would introduce solids into the infant's diet. Educational messages that highlighted this period, and the need to breastfeed more frequently, convinced mothers that solids were not yet necessary.

Avera Health System lactation specialist, Kathy English, who had been a leader in their mission teams since 2002, brought a lasting partnership to Haiti and improved our understanding and expertise in many ways. The teams that traveled from the numerous Avera health delivery centers brought experience and one-on-one training for the nurses and village health workers (*ajan de santé*).

Twice a year, the nurses, technicians, doctors, and pharmacists carried supplies to Haiti that supported the work of the HHF to advance exclusive breastfeeding; medicine cups for newborns, manual breast pumps, and electric models for the clinics, donations to purchase sippy cups for 6 month-olds, breast shields, 10 cc syringes to help mothers with inverted nipples, baby blankets, crocheted hats for newborns, and many other items. "Belly balls" and the breastfeeding baby mannequin were new to us, and effective teaching tools. Their concern and response to our need for assistance brought us to a much higher level of quality of care.

The volunteer nurses accompanied the Haitian nurse midwife for visits to the government hospital maternity unit. They helped new mothers and taught student nurses at the same time. They also donated educational and service supplies to the local nursing association and hospital nurse midwives. These actions further strengthened the Haitian Health Foundation partnership with the national nurses and local hospital.

International partnerships extended from service support to operation research beginning in 2005. The University of Connecticut School of Medicine faculty and students have helped HHF join science, practice, and experience with local realities to increase the exclusive breastfeeding rate from 1% to 80%, and to fundamentally change infant nutrition in rural Haitian villages. Medical and MPH students conducted 2-month projects answering questions in a systematic way to examine mothers' beliefs and knowledge, and recommend strategies to improve education, care, and monitoring.

In 2005, a nurse, who was an MPH student, examined HHF's monitoring of mother-infant feeding practices for the first 12 months postpartum. A notation was made on the woman's homebased health card as to whether she reported complete breastfeeding without return of menses, partial feeding, or token feeding. A monthly report of the mother was also documented on the computerized mother roster by the *ajan santé*. Selected home visits are made by nurse supervisors to confirm mother's reports. Use of the collected information was not uniform or consistent and the student recommendations are now standard practice for HHF. Routine practice in Haiti is primarily supportive counseling without monthly documentation (Roman, Susan (2007). *Exclusive breastfeeding practices in rural Haitian women.*

Master Thesis. Connecticut: University of Connecticut School of Medicine Public Health Program).

In 2006, a medical MPH student examined knowledge and practices of HIV positive mothers. One-hundred thirty four mothers were interviewed in the HHF referral center for maternal care Center of Hope. Women in the HHF service area (coverage of approximately 200,000 people) were significantly more knowledgeable about the benefits of exclusive breastfeeding than were women from outside of the HHF service area (Burcin Uygungil. (2006). *HIV and exclusive breastfeeding in Jeremie, Haiti.* Master's Thesis. University of Connecticut School of Medicine). Because of her study, educational messages were intensified at the institutional level so women not living in HHF areas would receive the same education about HIV and breastfeeding.

Spoiled-milk syndrome (*let gate*) is a condition when strong emotion causes breastmilk to mix with blood and be spoiled. It may go into the head. Special actions and teas are necessary to treat this condition. After the horrific earthquake in Port-au-Prince in January 2010, thousands of mothers and their babies returned, or came, to this area of Haiti. It was important to determine if, and how, mothers dealt with these emotions, loss of infrastructure, and availability of teas to treat *let gate*. A medical student interviewed breastfeeding women and collected their stories. Women used strategies such as drinking their own breastmilk to assure that it was safe. They continued feeding because there was no option of finding teas (Wonneberger, Kate. (2010). *Exclusive breastfeeding practices among post-earthquake migrants in rural Jeremie.* University of Connecticut Medical School, Farmington CT).

A recent student study about birth spacing in rural women found exclusive breastfeeding was an important factor. One-hundred and four Haitian women of reproductive age were interviewed about the spacing of their children. Concerning breastfeeding and family planning, 93% of women used Lactation Amenorrhea Method (LAM) at least once, 65% used it after every delivery, and 88% used it after at least half of their 383 deliveries (Gregorio, Leah. (2013, Summer). Determining factors associated with birth spacing of children in rural Haiti. Connecticut: University of Connecticut School of Medicine).

The partnerships described above are dynamic, ever-growing, and expanding. Moving forward, HHF has welcomed more than 10 organizations from all corners of Haiti to come to Jeremie to participate in breastfeeding education, support, documentation, and feedback. Often, counseling is the only approach used in Haiti to support immediate, exclusive, and sustained breastfeeding. The objectives of these field training experiences are to demonstrate what is possible in a low-resource setting. They participate with counterparts (nurse, *ajan santé*, community leaders, and traditional healers), discuss educational strategies, and collect HHF manuals, songs, and samples to bring home. They learn from the mothers themselves and plan a solid breastfeeding program for their own organization.

Without partnerships in the community, the region, the nation, and with international service and research colleagues, the Haitian Health Foundation could not have attained an exclusive breastfeeding rate of 80% for the first 6 months of life.

Building Partnerships at the State and National Levels for Breastfeeding-Friendly Childcare

Kathleen L. Anderson

Background

Breastfeeding support in the Early Care and Education (ECE) setting becomes increasingly more important as more women with children under the age of 1 year enter the work force (U.S. Department of Labor, 2013; U.S. Department of Health and Human Services, 2011). Most mothers desire to breastfeed their babies, as indicated by surveys of mothers' intentions, and by the number of women initiating breast-feeding (Centers for Disease Control, 2013; Declercq, Sakala, Corry, & Applebaum, 2006). A recent study, however, indicated that only 40% of mothers meet their breastfeeding goals (Odom, Li, Scanlon, Perrine, & Grummer-Strawn, 2013), and while some mothers in the work force are able to continue to breastfeed, most are not exclusively breastfeeding (Centers for Disease Control, 2013).

Returning to work after having a baby usually involves arranging for childcare, either with family members at home or out-of-the-home care. About half of all infants of working mothers are in out-of-home childcare settings (Kim & Peterson, 2008). Mothers cite returning to work, and using childcare, as reasons to stop breastfeeding. According to researchers, infants who are routinely cared for by someone other than their mothers are significantly less likely to be breastfed (Kim & Peterson, 2008).

The Surgeon General recognized the importance of the ECE provider for the success of the breastfeeding relationship (U.S. Department of Health and Human Services, 2011). The ECE setting was considered as one of the communities that had a role in supporting breastfeeding families, and Action 16 called ECE professionals to "ensure that all child care providers accommodate the needs of breastfeeding mothers and infants."

How are the states responding to the *Surgeon General's Call to Action* to meet the needs of breastfeeding families in the ECE setting? What partnerships already exist or need to be created to facilitate the implementation of statewide programs to support breastfeeding in childcare?

The National Collaborative for Advancing Breastfeeding in Childcare

The Carolina Global Breastfeeding Institute (CGBI) hosted the first meeting of the National Collaborative for Advancing Breastfeeding in Childcare, formerly the Interstate Collaboration on Breastfeeding Support in Child Care, with support from the W.K. Kellogg Foundation (WKKF), to examine these and other questions. Twenty-four participants, representing twelve states with statewide breastfeeding in childcare programs, or recent WKKF funding to develop programs, and two national organizations, met to discuss breastfeeding supportive childcare. It was the first time that representatives from states with statewide breastfeeding in childcare programs came together, and by gathering in one place, participants were able to increase awareness of each other's programs, and to discuss implementation and lessons learned during program implementation.

The primary goals of the working group meeting were to increase knowledge and understanding among the programs, explore best practices for supporting breastfeeding in the ECE setting, and to begin to develop collaboration and consensus on the factors associated with the challenges and opportunities for sustainable implementation of breastfeeding in childcare programs, and for widespread dissemination. Recommendations, in particular those for building state-national partnerships, will be presented here.

Partnerships for Implementation

The statewide programs for supporting breastfeeding in childcare represented a mix of coordination and partnership approaches to implementation and sustainability. Coordination was carried out by state agencies for half of the programs. However, five programs were coordinated by non-state organizations, and one through informal coordination that was not reflected in either a state agency or non-state organization classification. The majority of the states developed state and non-governmental partnerships for implementation and coordination, although two states built partnerships solely within state agencies, and two solely within non-governmental organizations.

Partnership for Consistency

State regulations provide essential benchmarks for determining program content of statewide programs to support breastfeeding in childcare. However, state regulations may not always follow best practice. State regulations often need to be updated, and may not be in step with national standards. For example, state regulations related to exclusive breastfeeding guidelines, and to human milk handling-and-storage guidelines, often are not consistent with national standards (e.g., Caring for Our Children National Health and Safety Performance Standards). There is a need for a platform for interchange, where states could develop consistent messaging without usurping the individual state's standards or regulations. Building a partnership of state and national representatives to explore current national standards could provide the opportunity to create consistent messaging for developing regulations throughout the county, while allowing flexibility for individual states to develop regulations based on these consistent messages. In addition, a state-national partnership could explore the effectiveness of providing breastfeeding-friendly childcare designations versus integrating standards directly into the national quality rating system (i.e., Quality Rating Improvement System [QRIS]).

Partnership for Resource Sharing

State/national partnerships provide opportunities for bringing together the large amount of experience and perspective inherent in the many statewide programs, as well as the variety of materials and resources. These partnerships could address issues related to resources and materials that might be barriers to implementation of statewide programs by developing common materials (e.g., toolkits) for dissemination nationally.

Partnership for Sustainability

A state/national partnership with representation from diverse fields, such as breastfeeding, public health, health care, childcare, disparities/equities, and early child development and education, would develop a more sustainable, consistent message for policy, certification, and accreditation. Who are the stakeholders in early childhood health and nutrition at the state and national levels? Potential stakeholders in a state/national partnership could include state and national agencies related to childcare licensing, certification, and accreditation, education, and breastfeeding. State/national partnerships also may include State CACFP and breastfeeding coalitions. These state/national partnerships would have the added purpose of bringing together governmental, and non-governmental, stakeholders who would be in positions to promote buy-in, and facilitate continued assessment and evaluation for sustainability of state programs to provide breastfeeding-friendly support in childcare.

Conclusions

More women with children under the age of 1 year are entering the workforce (U.S. Department of Health and Human Services, 2011; U.S. Department of Labor, 2013). Breastfeeding-supportive early care and education programs are vital components to "ensure that all childcare providers accommodate the needs of breastfeeding mothers and infants" (U.S. Department of Health and Human Services, 2011). State/national partnerships that bring together representatives from diverse disciplines can develop sustainable, consistent messages for breastfeeding-friendly childcare policy, certification, and accreditation. A national, consistent message would enable families to make appropriate early care and education choices that support their decisions to continue to breastfeed.

References

Centers for Disease Control and Prevention. (2013). Breastfeeding report card. United States. Retrieved from www.cdc.gov/breastfeeding/pdf/2013breastfeedingreportcard.pdf

Declercq, E., Sakala, C., Corry, M., & Applebaum, S. (2006). *Listening to mothers II: Report of the second national US survey of women's childbearing experiences*. New York: Childbirth Connection. Retrieved from www.childbirthconnection.org/article.asp?ck=10396

Kim, J. & Peterson, K. (2008). Association of infant child care with infant feeding practices and weight gain among US Infants. *Archives of Pediatrics and Adolescent Medicine, 162*(7), 627-633. doi:10.1001/archpedi.162.7.627

Odom, E. C., Li, R., Scanlon, K. S., Perrine, C. G., & Grummer-Strawn, L. (2013). Reasons for earlier than desired cessation of breastfeeding. *Pediatrics, 131*(3), e726-e732. doi: 10.1542/peds.2012-1295

U.S. Bureau of Labor Statistics, Department of Labor. (2013). Happy mother's day from Bureau of Labor Statistics: Working mothers in 2012. *The Editor's Desk.* Retrieved from http://www.bls.gov/opub/ted/2013/ted_20130510.htm

U.S. Department of Health and Human Services. (2011). *The Surgeon General's call to action to support breastfeeding.* Washington, DC: U.S. Department of Health and Human Services, Office of the Surgeon General.

Section Ic
State and Local Partnerships

CHAPTER 6

A Statewide Assessment of Worksite Lactation Support Programs—Georgia, 2013

Chinelo Ogbuanu, Theresa Chapple-McGruder,
Relda Robertson-Beckley, Evan Carey, and Seema Csukas

Introduction

Breastfeeding is recognized as the best way to feed most infants. The American Academy of Pediatrics [AAP] and other professional organizations in the United States recommend exclusive breastfeeding for the first 6 months of life (American Academy of Pediatrics, 2012; American College of Obstetricians and Gynecologists, 2007; American Dietetic Association, 2005). From age 6 months, the AAP recommends continuing breastfeeding, with supplementation with other foods for 1 year and beyond (American Academy of Pediatrics, 2012).

In the United States, more than 50% of mothers of infants participate in the work force (U.S. Bureau of Labor Statistics, 2011), and work-related issues have been cited as reasons for non-initiation (Ahluwalia, Morrow, & Hsia, 2005; Arora, McJunkin, Wehrer, & Kuhn, 2000; Guttman & Zimmerman, 2000; Khoury, Moazzem, Jarjoura, Carothers, & Hinton, 2005; Ogbuanu et al., 2009; Taylor, Risica, & Cabral, 2003), and early cessation of breastfeeding (Ahluwalia et al., 2005; Kimbro, 2006; Taylor et al., 2003). Recent reports (U.S. Department of Health and Human Services, 2008, 2011) clearly delineate the benefits of high-quality employer support for breast-feeding employees; better retention of experienced workers, higher employee morale, greater loyalty and productivity of employees, reduction in absenteeism and sick leave taken by parents of young children, and lower health care and health insurance costs.

Nationally, 25% of employers have lactation-support programs or provide an on-site lactation/mother's room (Society for Human Resources Management [SHRM], 2009). *The Healthy People (HP) 2020* goal is to increase the proportion of employers that have worksite lactation support programs (LSPs) to 38% (U.S. Department of Health and Human Services, 2010). The Patient Protection and Affordable Care Act (PPACA), signed into law in 2010, may provide the needed boost in attaining this goal. The PPACA amended Section 7 of the Fair Labor Standards Act of 1938. It requires that employers with 50 or more employees provide a reasonable break time as needed for an employee to express human milk for her nursing child in a private place other than the bathroom during the child's first year of life (Patient Protection and Affordable Care Act, 2010). Some state breastfeeding-friendly laws predate the PPACA. Georgia, for example, enacted a state worksite breastfeeding statute in 1999, second only to the state of Texas (Abdulloeva & Eyler, 2013). The Georgia law allows employers to provide daily unpaid break time for a mother to express human milk for her infant child ("Employer obligation to provide time for women to express human milk for infant child," 1999). The law also requires employers to make a reasonable effort to provide a private location other than a toilet stall in close proximity to the workplace for this activity. The employer is not required to provide break time if doing so would unduly disrupt the workplace operations.

Although the baseline proportion of LSPs in the nation is known, no such baseline exists in Georgia. To address this gap, we conducted a survey of major employers (50+ employees) in Georgia to assess the proportion that provide LSPs for their employees. We also examined the level of support and associated factors to the support provided.

Methods

We developed a breastfeeding-friendly worksite survey using ideas from the literature (Texas Department of State Health Services, 2011; U.S. Breastfeeding Committee, 2002, 2003, 2010; U.S. Department of Health and Human Services, 2008, 2011). Data collected includes company characteristics, policies, and facilities. We pilot-tested the survey in November 2012 among agencies housed in our building. The feedback from the pilot testing indicated that the survey questions were clear and could be completed within 15 minutes. Upon contracting with a survey research institute for survey fielding, another pilot testing was done by the institute, resulting in slight modifications to ambiguous questions based on respondent feedback. We targeted businesses with a verified or projected size of 50+ employees and a valid mailing or email address on file with the contracted research institute. Beginning in July 2013, surveys were sent to a random sample of 3,705 unique businesses from a database of 14, 835 unique businesses in Georgia. Surveys were sent via paper mail (1,250) and email (2,455). After a wait period of 3 weeks, phone calls were made to non-responders over a five-day period. Follow-up emails were then sent every two weeks through November 2013. The survey was finally closed in December 2013.

Following a review of the literature on needed worksite support for lactating mothers (Allen, Belay, & Perrine, 2014; Garvin et al., 2013; Marinelli, Moren, & Taylor, 2013; Murtagh & Moulton, 2011), we created a breastfeeding friendliness (BF) index from eight survey variables, namely; type of lactation room (dedicated [score =3], floating [2], other [1], none [0]), availability of paid maternity leave (1), availability of one or more return-to-work policies after maternity leave (1), provision of breastfeeding accommodations that allow women to breastfeed on site (1), availability of work breaks for women to breastfeed or express milk (1), presence of company support for breastfeeding employees, such as breastfeeding education, provision of skilled lactation care providers, etc. (1), agreement with the statement, "My company is supportive of breastfeeding" (1), and whether the company makes breast pumps available to employees (1). The BF index ranged from 0 to10 and was categorized as low (0 to 3), medium (4 to 6), and high (7 to10).

After the data was cleaned, descriptive analysis was conducted on all variables. Bivariate analysis between selected company characteristics and the BF index was conducted. Since the outcome, BF index, was a 3-level variable with ordered categories (low, medium, and high), we conducted a multinomial logistic regression using the cumulative logit approach. We modeled the outcome, BF index, on selected company characteristics (company size: small [0 to 49 employees], medium [50 to 499], and large [≥500]; city size of business location: [population of <100, 000 and ≥100,000]; number of years in existence [≤30 and >30 years]; percent of female employees employed full-time [≤50%, >50%]; and percent of female employees of childbearing age [0-25%, 26-50%, >50%]). Alpha was set at 0.05. All analyses were performed using SAS 9.2. This study was approved in accordance with expedited ethical review procedures by the Georgia Department of Public Health Institutional Review Board.

Results

Descriptive

A total of 280 businesses completed the survey (210 responses via paper mail, 51 via email, 19 by phone, overall response rate = 7.6%). Among those who completed the survey, the average business size was 879 employees, with a median of 90 employees (range: 2 to 80,000). Twenty-eight percent of businesses were small, 46% were mid-sized, 13% were large, and 13% were missing information on business size. About 65% of businesses had more than 50% of their female employees employed full-time. Thirty-four percent of businesses had 0 to 25% of their female employees in the childbearing age range (15 to 44 years), 35% had 26% to 50%, and 28% had more than 50% of their female employees in the childbearing age range. Thirty-four percent of businesses were located in cities with a population size of < 100,000, 49% in cities of ≥100,000, and 17% were missing information on city size. The average length of time for which businesses had been in existence was 44 years, with a median of 30 years (range: 2 to 200 years). About half (155 [55%]) of the businesses provided a space (other than a restroom) for breastfeeding or expressing human milk. The space varied as follows: dedicated:16.8%; floating: 27.5%; other: 10.4%; none: 33.2%; and missing: 12.1%. The median BF index was 5.0. The BF index was almost evenly distributed (30%-low, 40%-medium, 30%-high).

Bivariate and Multivariate Analyses

In the bivariate analysis, business size ($p=0.0016$), and city size where business is located ($p=0.002$) were positively associated the BF index. Adjusted analysis using multinomial logistic regression revealed that large businesses, when compared to small businesses, had more than 6 times greater odds of having a higher versus lower BF index category (OR=6.44; 95% CI:2.44-16.95). In addition, businesses located in cities with a population size of ≥ 100,000 compared to those located in cities with a population size of < 100,000 had more than twice the odds of having a higher versus lower BF index category (OR=2.36; 95% CI:1.38-4.05). Even though the estimates were positive for all other variables in the model, none other reached statistical significance.

Discussion

In summary, approximately half of the businesses sampled meet the Fair Labor Standards Act requirement of having a space (other than a restroom) for expressing human milk, but less than one-fifth have a dedicated breastfeeding space. About a third of the businesses had a high BF index. Adjusted analysis showed that business and city size were associated with breastfeeding friendliness. Similar to our findings, the 2009 Employee Benefits survey conducted by the Society for Human Resources Management (SHRM) showed that large organizations (≥500) were most likely to offer many family-friendly benefits (Society for Human Resources Management, 2009). For example, even though, overall, 25% of the companies surveyed provided an on-site lactation/mother's room, the distribution by company size was as follows: small (1 to 99 employees):12%; medium (100 to 499 employees): 26%; large (≥500 employees): 38% (Society for Human Resources Management, 2009).

The findings from our study are applicable to only the businesses who responded. Our study was limited by the low response rate and relatively small sample size. This may have led to a non-response bias. We wonder whether the low response rate could be attributable to our wording of the informed consent document, which was very explicit as to the voluntary nature of participation. In addition, we did not offer any incentives for participation. We only promised to share aggregated results with the participants, and we provided a number to call for technical assistance in developing or improving the company's breastfeeding support policy. The 2009 Employee Benefit survey conducted by the SHRM yielded a response rate of 19% (Society for Human Resources Management, 2009). This higher RR may be due to the fact that the benefit survey was sent to a sample of member businesses. The respondents may have felt some obligation to respond to the survey since they belonged to the society.

Although we targeted businesses with 50 or more employees, our final study sample included businesses with less than 50 employees. This may be attributed to the fact that the responses on business size were based on the respondents' knowledge and may not have been accurate. In addition, as earlier stated, some businesses in the database had a projected sample size based on an algorithm used by the research institute. This projection, which informed the sampling procedures, may also have been inaccurate. However, the presence of small businesses in our sample gave us the opportunity to explore how small businesses fared regarding provision of LSPs for their employees. It is also worthy of note that small businesses are not automatically exempt from fulfilling the requirements of the PPACA, as they need to demonstrate hardship to be exempted (Murtagh & Moulton, 2011; "Patient Protection and Affordable Care Act," 2010).

Findings from this study will help with targeting technical assistance in developing state-of-the-art LSPs and in establishing breastfeeding-friendly worksites in Georgia. Future research may assess differences, if any, between responders and non-responders, and elicit other explanatory variables of worksite breastfeeding friendliness.

References

Abdulloeva, S., & Eyler, A. A. (2013). Policies on worksite lactation support within states and organizations. *Journal of Women's Health (Larchmont)*, *22*(9), 769-774. doi: 10.1089/jwh.2012.4186

Ahluwalia, I. B., Morrow, B., & Hsia, J. (2005). Why do women stop breastfeeding? Findings from the Pregnancy Risk Assessment and Monitoring System. *Pediatrics, 116*(6), 1408-1412.

Allen, J. A., Belay, B., & Perrine, C. G. (2014). Using mPINC data to measure breastfeeding support for hospital employees. *Journal of Human Lactation, 30*(1), 97-101. doi: 0890334413495974

American Academy of Pediatrics. (2012). Breastfeeding and the use of human milk. *Pediatrics, 129*(3), e827-e841. doi: 10.1542/peds.2011-3552

American College of Obstetricians and Gynecologists. (2007). ACOG Committee Opinion No. 361: Breastfeeding: maternal and infant aspects. *Obstetrics & Gynecology, 109*(2 Pt 1), 479-480.

American Dietetic Association. (2005). Position of the American Dietetic Association: Promoting and supporting breastfeeding. *Journal American Dietitic Association, 105*(5), 810-818.

Arora, S., McJunkin, C., Wehrer, J., & Kuhn, P. (2000). Major factors influencing breastfeeding rates: Mother's perception of father's attitude and milk supply. *Pediatrics, 106*(5), E67.

Garvin, C. C., Sriraman, N. K., Paulson, A., Wallace, E., Martin, C. E., & Marshall, L. (2013). The business case for breastfeeding: A successful regional implementation, evaluation, and follow-up. *Breastfeeding Medicine, 8*(4), 413-417. doi: 10.1089/bfm.2012.0104

Guttman, N. & Zimmerman, D. R. (2000). Low-income mothers' views on breastfeeding. *Social Science and Medicine, 50*(10), 1457-1473.

Khoury, A. J., Moazzem, S. W., Jarjoura, C. M., Carothers, C., & Hinton, A. (2005).

Breastfeeding initiation in low-income women: Role of attitudes, support, and perceived control. *Women's Health Issues, 15*(2), 64-72.

Kimbro, R. T. (2006). On-the-job moms: Work and breastfeeding initiation and duration for a sample of low-income women. *Maternal Child Health Journal, 10*(1), 19-26.

Marinelli, K. A., Moren, K., & Taylor, J. S. (2013). Breastfeeding support for mothers in workplace employment or educational settings: Summary statement. *Breastfeeding Medicine, 8*(1), 137-142. doi: 10.1089/bfm.2013.9999

Murtagh, L., & Moulton, A. D. (2011). Working mothers, breastfeeding, and the law. *American Journal of Public Health, 101*(2), 217-223. doi: AJPH.2009.185280

Ogbuanu, C. A., Probst, J., Laditka, S. B., Liu, J., Baek, J., & Glover, S. (2009). Reasons why women do not initiate breastfeeding: A southeastern state study. *Women's Health Issues, 19*(4), 268-278. doi: S1049-3867(09)00030-9

Patient Protection and Affordable Care Act, Pub. L. No. P.L. 111-148 § Sec. 4207 (2010).

Society for Human Resources Management (SHRM). (2009). *2009 Employee benefits: A survey report by the Society for Human Resource Management.* United States of America. Retrieved from http://www.shrm.org/research/surveyfindings/articles/documents/09-0295_employee_benefits_survey_report_spread_fnl.pdf

Taylor, J. S., Risica, P. M., & Cabral, H. J. (2003). Why primiparous mothers do not breastfeed in the United States: A national survey. *Acta Paediatrica, 92*(11), 1308-1313.

Texas Department of State Health Services. (2011). *Texas Mother-Friendly Business Application*. Retrieved September 29, 2011, from https://www.dshs.state.tx.us/wichd/lactate/mfwapp.shtm

U.S. Bureau of Labor Statistics, Department of Labor. (2011). Employment characteristics of families—2010. *The Editor's Desk*. Retrieved from http://www.bls.gov/opub/ted/2011/ted_20110328.htm

U.S. Department of Health and Human Services. (2011). *The Surgeon General's call to action to support breastfeeding*. Washington, DC: Department of Health and Human Services, Office of the Surgeon General. Retrieved from http://www.surgeongeneral.gov/library/calls/breastfeeding/calltoactiontosupportbreastfeeding.pdf

U.S. Breastfeeding Committee. (2002). *Workplace breastfeeding support* [Issue paper]. Raleigh, NC: United States Breastfeeding Committee. Retrieved from http://www.usbreastfeeding.org/Portals/0/Publications/Workplace-2002-USBC.pdf

U.S. Breastfeeding Committee. (2003). *Accommodations for breastfeeding in the workplace*. Washington, DC: United States Breastfeeding Committee. Retrieved from http://www.usbreastfeeding.org/Portals/0/Publications/Workplace-Checklist-2002-USBC.pdf

U.S. Breastfeeding Committee. (2010). *Workplace accommodations to support and protect breastfeeding*. Washington, DC: United States Breastfeeding Committee.

U.S. Department of Health and Human Services. (2010). MICH-22 Increase the proportion of employers that have worksite lactation support programs. *Healthy People 2020*. Retrieved from http://www.healthypeople.gov/2020/topicsobjectives2020/TechSpecs.aspx?hp2020id=MICH-22

U.S. Department of Health and Human Services. (2008). *The Business Case for Breastfeeding*. Rockville, MD: Health Resources and Services Administration.

North Carolina Breastfeeding Coalition: Working Together for Change

Kathy Parry

The North Carolina Breastfeeding Coalition (NCBC) is a nonprofit organization bringing together health care providers, agencies, organizations, individuals, families, and all other breast-feeding advocates to promote, protect, and support breastfeeding in the state of North Carolina. Inclusion of varied stakeholders is vital to the continual expansion of the landscape of breastfeeding support for mothers. This work is an ongoing and ever-evolving process requiring good communication strategies.

Founded in 2005, the organization's vision is to ensure that exclusive and continued breastfeeding is the norm in North Carolina. NCBC provides a framework for the development and implementation of programs to advance breastfeeding support throughout North Carolina. In addition, NCBC provides a forum for creation and exchange of resources for breastfeeding professionals and families. The organization's volunteers also help women advocate for themselves should they have grievances related to breastfeeding at work or in public.

NCBC Project Descriptions and Partners

Table 1 lists several current projects of NCBC and details the partners engaged in each. Added descriptions of selected projects are included below the table. In addition to these partners, we actively collaborate with the United States Breastfeeding Committee, and the North Carolina Division of Public Health, both of which are described later.

NCBC Projects	Partners/Advocates
Ban the Bags (Golden Bow Award)	National Alliance for Breastfeeding Advocacy (NABA) Public Citizen Maternity Centers in North Carolina North Carolina Division of Public Health UNC School of Public Health students
Business Case for Breastfeeding Awards	Human Resources and Services Administration (HRSA) North Carolina Division of Public Health Businesses in North Carolina UNC School of Public Health students
Donor Human Milk Awareness	North Carolina State University students Families of North Carolina Wake Med Mothers Milk Bank University of North Carolina Maternal and Child Health Students
IBLCE Exam Scholarships	Aspiring Internationally Board Certified Lactation Consultants in North Carolina
Licensure of IBCLCs	North Carolina Lactation Consultant Association North Carolina State Legislature North Carolina Child Fatality Task Force Carolina Global Breastfeeding Institute at UNC School of Public Health
Medicaid Reimbursement	North Carolina Lactation Consultant Association North Carolina State Legislature North Carolina Child Fatality Task Force Carolina Global Breastfeeding Institute at UNC School of Public Health
Mini-Grant Funding Awards	North Carolina organizations that support breastfeeding
Outreach	Local breastfeeding coalitions in North Carolina Community members in North Carolina

Ban the Bags (Golden Bow Award)

The National Alliance for Breastfeeding Advocacy (NABA) maintains a website highlighting the importance of eliminating marketing of infant formula in maternity centers. When we award facilities in North Carolina who have successfully banned the formula discharge bags, we send them the link and encourage them to register their facility so that they can be included in the national effort. Registration must be done by individual facilities. Students from both North Carolina State University and the UNC School of Public Health contribute to the Golden Bow Award efforts by reaching out to hospital contacts to inform them about the campaign. The North Carolina Division of Public Health also promotes the Golden Bow Award through the NC Maternity Center Breastfeeding-Friendly Designation (NC MCBFD) which is a state recognition program based on the *Ten Steps to Successful Breastfeeding*. Step six includes banning formula discharge bags in hospitals.

Public Citizen is a national nonprofit organization dedicated to protecting health, safety, and democracy. According to their recent study, the vast majority of the top-ranked US hospitals have stopped distributing bags with formula samples to new mothers. A follow-up report highlights varied successful initiatives from 11 specific states, including North Carolina. The states of Rhode Island and Massachusetts are completely bag-free, and North Carolina is working toward similar achievement: more than 82% of live births in North Carolina occur in maternity centers free from infant-formula marketing.

Business Case for Breastfeeding Awards

The U.S. Health Resources and Services Administration (HRSA), together with the Department of Health and Human Services, the Maternal and Child Health Bureau and the Office of Women's Health supported efforts to help states implement the Business Case for Breastfeeding in 2009. Central to this effort was the free distribution of toolkits for employers detailing how to achieve a breastfeeding-friendly worksite, while achieving return on this investment. North Carolina was fortunate to benefit from this initial funding stream, which included a two-day training for coalition members and public health partners, and facilitated the launch of our current program that awards businesses for achieving simple milestones toward supporting breastfeeding employees and/or customers. Students from the UNC School of Public Health, under the guidance of the Carolina Global Breastfeeding Institute, help make businesses across the state aware of the awards.

NCBC collaborated with two branches of the NC Division of Public Health to develop and disseminate a state-specific document detailing how North Carolina businesses can become more supportive of breastfeeding. Now in its 2nd edition, *Eat Smart, Move More NC: Businesses Leading the Way in Support of Breastfeeding*, is a planning and resource guide for employers in North Carolina that outlines federal and state breastfeeding-related mandates, and shares success stories from North Carolina. NCBC continues to award businesses semi-annually with a plaque and window cling that states, "Breastfeeding Welcome Here."

Donor Human Milk Awareness

Increasing awareness of the benefits of utilizing donor human milk, as well as increasing the availability of donor human milk, are two essential goals for improving optimal health of neonates unable to receive a full supply of their mother's own milk. NCBC collaborated with students from North Carolina State University, under the guidance of Assistant Professor of Nutrition, Dr. April Fogleman, to develop brochures about donor milk with two distinct messages: one for increasing the demand for use of donor milk when supplementation is needed, and one for increasing the number of women choosing to donate their milk to the Wake Med Mothers Milk Bank.

United States Breastfeeding Committee

The United States Breastfeeding Committee (USBC) is an independent nonprofit coalition of more than 50 nationally influential professional, educational, and governmental organizations that share a common mission to drive collaborative efforts for policy and practices that create a landscape of breastfeeding support across the United States. Through the technical assistance of the USBC, all 50 states have formed breastfeeding coalitions. These coalitions are integral to mobilizing state and local efforts to promote breastfeeding. Coalitions have representation at USBC's membership meetings via two elected representatives that represent each distinct region.

The support of USBC has been a primary facilitator in enhancing the capacity of NCBC to initiate programs. NCBC has applied for, and been awarded, several grants that have helped to establish sustainable programs in the state of North Carolina. USBC offers technical assistance for these grants or subcontracts, which has proven vital for the development of the programs. In addition to financial and technical assistance, USBC hosts bi-monthly webinars for all state coalitions for information sharing and inspiration. Following each bi-monthly webinar, USBC hosts a regional call for leaders of coalitions among regions. These calls provide the space to share with, and learn from, other nearby coalitions and discuss challenges.

North Carolina Division of Public Health

Developing a relationship with a state health department is a vital step for any state breastfeeding coalition. There may be more than one branch that would be relevant for state coalition work, such as women's and children's services and nutrition, or their equivalent. The state health department may have funds available that could be allocated for breastfeeding advocacy and support.

The state of North Carolina is very supportive of breastfeeding and offers a number of resources for breastfeeding advocates. The work of NCBC is often in close collaboration with efforts at the North Carolina Division of Public Health (NCDPH). As such, the North Carolina State Breastfeeding Coordinator serves as an ex-officio member on the NCBC board.

NCBC has helped in the dissemination of several seminal resources coming out of the state office, including *Promoting, Protecting and Supporting Breastfeeding: A North Carolina Blueprint for Action* (2006), *Blueprint Status Report: Promoting, Protecting and Supporting Breastfeeding in North Carolina* (2011), and *Eat Smart North Carolina: Businesses Leading the Way in Support of Breastfeeding* (2010 and 2013 update). In addition, the coalition helped in the development of the latter document. NCBC also actively promotes NCDPH's two breastfeeding-friendly designation programs; the NC MCBFD and the North Carolina Breastfeeding-Friendly Childcare Designation. Two NCBC members are appointed to serve on the review committee for the NC MCBFD.

Coalition Membership and Action

State breastfeeding coalitions are most often volunteer-based organizations. As such, community membership is critical to carrying out and sustaining any projects or programs the coalition is able to implement. The funding for coalition initiatives may be from "soft money," or grants/subcontracts, which means that the organization requires another stream of funds to maintain any non-funded projects, as well as to sustain its basic operations. An annual donation for membership to a state breastfeeding coalition is one way that breastfeeding advocates can help contribute to the continued growth of the availability of support for breastfeeding mothers in their state. Dedicating skills and time is another way to contribute. Many minds make for better projects/initiatives, and many hands make for light work. As Margaret Mead once said: "Never doubt that a small group of thoughtful, committed citizens can change the world. Indeed, it is the only thing that ever has."

Resources

- http://ncbfc.org/
- http://www.usbreastfeeding.org/
- http://www.banthebags.org/
- http://www.citizen.org/documents/Best-Hospitals-End-Infant-Formula-Marketing-to-Support-Breastfeeding-Report.pdf
- http://www.citizen.org/documents/report-successful-initiatives-formula-marketing.pdf

Forging Partnerships for Breastfeeding in Richmond, Virginia

Rose Stith-Singleton, Cecilia E. Barbosa,
Leslie Lytle, Kellie E. Carlyle, Saba W. Masho

Introduction

The low rate of breastfeeding is a major public health problem that requires immediate attention. The benefits of breastfeeding in reducing infant and maternal morbidities are widely recognized (Allen & Hector, 2005; Hah-Holbrook, Haselton, Schetter, & Glynn, 2013; Sipsma, Magriples, Divney, Gordon, Gabzdyl, & Kershaw, 2013; Watkins, Meltzer-Brody, Zolnoun, & Stuebe, 2011; World Health Organization, 2013). The American Academy of Pediatrics recommends that infants be breastfed, or receive human milk, without supplemental foods or fluids for the first 6 months of life (Centers for Disease Control and Prevention, 2009). Despite its benefits, the majority of low-income women do not breastfeed (American Academy of Pediatrics, 2010). This problem is even more accentuated among low-income women who are recipients of the federally funded special supplemental nutrition program for Women, Infants, and Children (WIC). In 2011, only 4.3% of Richmond WIC participants selected the full WIC breastfeeding package, which is much lower than the national average of 11.2% (U.S. Department of Agriculture/Food and Nutrition Services, 2012). Recognizing the problem, the Mayor of Richmond charged the local Richmond Healthy Start Initiative (RHSI) to mobilize the community and increase the number of women who breastfeed their children. With that charge, Richmond City became the first locality in Virginia to establish a Mayor's Breastfeeding Commission, part of a broader Healthy Richmond Campaign. Richmond City was also the first to bring together business, government, and health care advocates to address this issue.

The RHSI is a federally funded initiative whose members have extensive experience working with low-income and underserved communities in Richmond City. Currently, the RHSI has over 100 member stakeholders working under the umbrella of the RHSI consortium. Members of the consortium are committed to improving the health of women and children. In the past two decades, the RHSI has made significant strides in reducing racial disparities in perinatal health. Most of its success was due to its ability to mobilize and engage an array of diverse stakeholders to achieve its goals. Notably, the charges for breastfeeding given to the RHSI emanated from the initiative's longstanding trusting relationship with the community and its track record in mobilizing the community.

The Mayor's Breastfeeding Commission

The RHSI utilized its experience with the consortium to establish the Mayor's Breastfeeding Commission. Commission members comprised a diverse group of leaders from the public, private non-profit, education, business, and community sectors, specifically chosen to reflect a wide range of expertise and experience. Diversity in terms of demographics, professional expertise, and community representation was consciously cultivated so that Commission members could lead breastfeeding promotion within multiple spheres of influence.

In forming the Commission, stakeholders were contacted individually and informed of the Mayor's charges. This stage was the most important step in the creation of a successful commission. Efforts were made to provide data informing stakeholders of the magnitude of the problem and drew upon the Centers for Disease Control and Prevention's evidence-based recommendations (Centers for Disease Control and Prevention, 2014). These documents were shared and discussed at individual stakeholder meetings. This process was the foundation for obtaining buy-in from stakeholders and ensuring lasting commitments.

The individual meetings were followed by a large Breastfeeding Commission meeting where Mayor Dwight C. Jones presented his charges and obtained input from members. As a result, the Commission was charged with three important goals: (1) increase breastfeeding rates in the City, especially among underserved, fragile women; (2) develop and implement a comprehensive multifaceted initiative with promise in increasing breastfeeding numbers; and (3) develop a social marketing campaign to increase citizen awareness and knowledge regarding the benefits of breastfeeding, including access to resources.

Commission Processes

The Commission met monthly from July 2011 until July 2012. Commission members received a Resource Notebook with information compiled from the Centers for Disease Control and Prevention's, *Guide to Breastfeeding Interventions* (Centers for Disease Control and Prevention, 2014), *Surgeon's General's Call to Action to Support Breastfeeding* (U.S. Department of Health and Human Services, 2011), and Health Resources and Services Administration's, *Business Case for Breastfeeding* (U.S. Department of Health and Human Services, 2014). Workgroups were formed, focused on the following areas; Health Care Providers (providers of direct pre-conception and perinatal care in public health, private practice, or community health settings); Community Educators/Programs (individuals or representatives of organizations that primarily provide services within the community or home setting); Business Case for Breastfeeding (representatives from the business community who may assist in the design or utilization of policies and procedures that facilitate lactation in the work setting); Hospital Community (representatives of hospital facilities and individuals who provide care directly or indirectly in hospital settings); and Social Media (commission members with expertise and/or interest in social media campaigns). These workgroups developed recommendations that were then vetted in public forums, and ultimately distilled down to four basic recommendations: (1) encourage Richmond health systems to adopt the 10 Steps of the Baby-Friendly Hospital Initiative to achieve the 2020 Healthy People Goals; (2) support and encourage Richmond City businesses to develop and implement comprehensive lactation support programs for their employees and patrons; (3) promote partnerships and education among care providers who come into contact with mothers, fathers, partners, and families before, during, and after childbirth, and during the infant's first year of life; and (4) develop an education/marketing strategy to promote breastfeeding. The final Commission recommendations were presented to and accepted by the Mayor in July of 2013.

Commission Successes in Community-Building

During the vetting period, Richmond Healthy Start Initiative utilized preliminary Commission recommendations to apply for a two-year Healthy Communities Action Team (HCAT) grant funded by the Virginia Foundation for Healthy Youth, which it received in July of 2012. Through this grant, a community coalition, the Richmond Health Action Alliance (RHAA), was formed. The RHAA-HCAT seeks to reduce childhood obesity in the City of Richmond through policy, infrastructure, and environmental changes that promote a breastfeeding-friendly and physically active community. The RHAA-HCAT was the primary sponsor of the 2013 Big Latch On and will again lead the 2014 Big Latch On.

In January of 2014, members of the Breastfeeding Commission were formally invited to participate in the RHAA-HCAT. This emerging coalition is actively engaged in building organizational and community alliances, and exploring opportunities to fulfill the Commission recommendations. Richmond Healthy Start Initiative recently received a two-year extension of the HCAT grant to continue its work in this area. As of this writing, one hospital system is close to completing the process of achieving the Baby-Friendly status, and another competing hospital has begun the process. During the summer of 2014, the coalition is piloting a Breastfeeding Ambassador Pilot Program in which 14 members of the African American and Hispanic communities will receive evidence-based lactation educator training and develop strategies for disseminating breastfeeding information into the community. In addition, five public awareness events are planned that will utilize the Breastfeeding Ambassadors as volunteer staff.

In parallel, Commission members from RHSI and Virginia Commonwealth University (VCU) secured a community-engagement grant from VCU to conduct 11 focus groups, and a survey among African American women who receive WIC benefits. The purpose of this collaborative initiative is to identify and understand the barriers and facilitators to infant feeding among these women, with an aim to inform the strategies of the RHAA-HCAT.

Conclusion

The Commission's work spawned initiatives to increase breastfeeding, including the establishment of the RHAA-HCAT; he previously described academic-community engagement research partnership to study barriers and facilitators to infant feeding among low-income African American women through focus groups and surveys of WIC participants; two lactation rooms in city government; progress by two hospital systems to become baby-friendly; and significant media attention to, and growing participation in, the Big Latch-On campaigns of 2012 and 2013 that were sponsored by RHSI with the support of all hospital systems.

RHSI, as leader of the Commission, was seen as a neutral and non-threatening party, capable of bringing together competing health systems, business representatives, and community members. Essential to successful collaboration was the Commission leaders' continual recognition of all members as valuable, knowledgeable, and experienced contributors who, in turn, fostered mutual respect among members. By creating a Resource Notebook and dedicating time at each meeting to joint learning, Commission leaders facilitated a common knowledge base among members. Another key component of its success was the high-level leadership involvement during the initial stages of the Commission. This included the presence of senior level management from three large competing health care systems serving Richmond (Virginia Commonwealth University, Bon Secours, and Hospital Corporation of America-HCA), the Chamber of Commerce, and the Virginia Department of Health at the kick-off press conference of the Commission. Having high-level multi-sector support at the kick-off set the tone for collaboration and engagement among Commission members.

Successfully creating the conditions for women to breastfeed requires a multi-sector approach with representation by diverse stakeholders. Involving multiple sectors (e.g., business, health care, media, government, community groups, and parents) from the beginning helped members understand and appreciate each other's roles and contributions. As the relationships among members developed, other collaborative partnerships emerged that facilitated both members and their home organizations promoting the goals and strategies of the Commission.

The Mayor's Breastfeeding Commission set in motion and continues to be a catalyst for community initiatives to raise breastfeeding rates. While much work remains, the involvement of high-level leadership, multi-sector, and diverse stakeholder representation, and collaborative engagement among members were essential for generating such early successes.

References

Allen, J., & Hector, D. (2005). Benefits of breastfeeding. *New South Wales Public Health Bulletin, 16*(4), 42- 46.

American Academy of Pediatrics. (2010). *Early breastfeeding initiation.* Retrieved from http://www2.aap.org/breastfeeding/Centers for Disease Control and Prevention. (2009). *Breastfeeding.* Retrieved from http://www.cdc.gov/breastfeeding/research/index.htm

Centers for Disease Control and Prevention. (2014). *The CDC guide to strategies to support breastfeeding mothers and babies.* Retrieved from http://www.cdc.gov/breastfeeding/resources/guide.htm

Hah-Holbrook, J., Haselton, M. G., Schetter, C. D., & Glynn, L. M. (2013). Does breastfeeding offer protection against maternal depressive symptomatology? *Archives of Women's Mental Health, 16,* 411-422.

Sipsma, H. L., Magriples, U., Divney, A., Gordon, D., Gabzdyl, E., & Kershaw, T. (2013). Breastfeeding behavior among adolescents: Initiation, duration, and exclusivity. *Journal of Adolescent Health, 53*(3), 394-400.

U.S. Department of Agriculture/Food and Nutrition Services, Supplemental Food Programs Division. (2012). *WIC breastfeeding data local agency report. FY 2011.* Retrieved from http://www.fns.usda.gov/sites/default/files/FY2010-BFdata-localagencyreport.pdf

U.S. Department of Health and Human Services. (2011). *The Surgeon General's call to action to support breastfeeding.* Washington, DC: U.S. Department of Health and Human Services, Office of the Surgeon General.

U.S. Department of Health and Human Services, Health Resources and Services Administration. (2014). *Business case for breastfeeding.* Retrieved from http://mchb.hrsa.gov/pregnancyandbeyond/breastfeeding/Watkins, S., Meltzer-Brody, S., Zolnoun, D., & Stuebe, A. (2011). Early breastfeeding experiences and postpartum depression. *Obstetrics & Gynecology, 118*(2, Part 1), 214-221.

World Health Organization. (2013). *Breastfeeding.* Retrieved from http://www.who.int/topics/breastfeeding/en/

Forging partnerships with Diverse Communities to Reduce Disparities in Breastfeeding and Increase Equity in Outcomes

Chapters in this section addresses the challenges of common messaging —breastfeeding—across diverse cultural and racial populations. The first paper addresses the underlying issues, while the next two address issues encountered by the African American mother, followed by two considering immigrant communities. Three papers addressing the challenges of LGBTQ parenting are followed by the special issue of breastfeeding among incarcerated women.

Section II a
Challenges of Race/Ethnicity, Culture, Class, Immigrant Status, and Power

Challenges of Multidisciplinary Breastfeeding Education: Culture, Class, and Power

Amanda L. Watkins and Joan E. Dodgson

Breastfeeding education for multi-disciplinary health care providers has long been advocated as effective in improving breastfeeding support and duration rates (Bernaix, Schmidt, Arrizola, Iovinelli, & Medina-Poelinez, 2008; Chezem, Friesen, & Parker, 2004; Declercq, Labbok, Sakala, & O'Hara, 2009; Hillenbrand & Larsen, 2002; Ingram, 2006; Ogburn, Espey, Leeman, & Alvarez, 2005; Renfrew, McFadden, Dykes et al. 2006; Smale, Renfrew, Marshall, & Spiby, 2006).Increasing knowledge of health care providers who work with breastfeeding families has been the focus of most efforts to improve in-hospital and community services for these families. Throughout the country, hospitals, state health departments, and clinics have spent a lot of money improving knowledge levels. Yet practices have been slow to change (DiGirolamo, Grummer-Strawn, & Fein, 2008). Why? The more we learn about the complexity of changing institutional practices, the clearer it becomes that practice change involves multi-dimensional levels of change at individual and structural (e.g., policy, procedures, administrative support) levels. The Baby-Friendly Hospital Initiative has successfully addressed these multi-dimensional levels (Chin, Myers, & Magnus, 2008; Criscco-Lizza, 2006). This is not a viable alternative for all hospitals. However, every hospital and community agency does have the responsibility to use best practices when caring for breastfeeding families.

Having a staff of health care providers knowledgeable about best practices is a necessary component of providing quality evidence-based lactation services, but not sufficient to create these services (DiGirolamo et al., 2008). Promoting knowledge acquisition as the primary strategy for changing practice fails to consider the structural and functional issues within agencies serving breastfeeding families, some of which are shared by hospital and community agencies and some are uniquely different. It is our thesis that the intersection of race, class, and employers' power structures provide the contextual ground for challenges faced when conducting breastfeeding education for health care providers, and for multidisciplinary learners.

For the past four years, we have been conducting multidisciplinary breastfeeding education programs for health care providers (physicians, nurses, dietitians, midwives, child-life specialists, and speech pathologists), and paraprofessional health care providers (WIC staff, doulas, childbirth educators, peer counselors, and medical assistants). Usually, we have slightly more paraprofessionals in attendance. Our programs have been required of WIC staff, primarily Latina, and of Indian Health Services staff throughout North Central Arizona. Through routine pre- and post-testing, we have repeatedly demonstrated effectiveness in transferring breastfeeding related knowledge for both professionals and paraprofessional participants. If knowledge acquisition was the only learning outcome measured, as it is in many studies, differences between course participants who were professionals and paraprofessional would not have emerged. Perhaps the frequent use of knowledge acquisition as the only measured learning outcome has contributed to the commonly held belief that targeting both professionals and paraprofessionals for the same educational programs is appropriate.

When educational outcomes beyond knowledge acquisition are desired, including professionals and paraprofessionals in the same classes may not be the most effective approach. Intention to perform breastfeeding supportive behaviors, and participants' perceived control over their breastfeeding practices, also have been measured with some positive changes occurring between the pre/post-test, which varied by cultural-orientation, social class, and status in work environment (professional/paraprofessional). In our research on measures of participants' ability to implement what was learned in class and ability to act independently to provide best practices, paraprofessionals scored much lower than professionals. Often paraprofessional participants perceived an inability to influence practice within their work environments, and reported that their work environments did not support breastfeeding women. The perceived lack of agency reported by paraprofessional participants reflects their socioeconomic status, educational backgrounds, and status within work setting, which were markedly differentiated in our sample. It is likely that these class and power differentials are found frequently across the country between professionals and paraprofessionals.

Cultural relevance, participants' education and reading levels, and voluntary vs. employer mandated class attendance can contribute to actual or perceived inequalities between professionals and paraprofessionals. Too often, designing breastfeeding education programs have lacked cultural relevance for participants. Educational outcomes are improved when the education has cultural relevance (Curley & Li, 2003; Ford & Airhihenbuwa, 2010; Grywacz, McMahan, Hurley, Stokols, & Phillips, 2004). Indeed, it is possible that the success reported by peer-to-peer support programs is in part due to cultural relevance provided by peers of the same cultural orientation.

In our classes, most professionals were Caucasian, and most paraprofessionals were minority women (i.e., Latina, Asian, and Native American). We have threaded cultural influences and relevant approaches throughout our program. While the diversity of our participants has provided opportunities for cross-cultural discussions, it is possible that the social status differentials within the group deterred some minority women from actively participating in these discussions. Providing separate educational programs for professionals and paraprofessional would provide an opportunity to test this hypothesis.

It is important to tailor educational materials to the reading level of class participants. This can be a problem when a large gap occurs in the education levels of class participants. We require participants to read large portions of a popular basic lactation textbook. The WIC and Indian Health Service agencies we have worked with have been very supportive and provided participants from their agencies with copies of this text. However, many of the paraprofessionals are immigrants, with lower reading levels than the professionals, and struggle with the content and amount of reading. The extra work that English-as-a-second-language (ESL) students have to do to keep up with non-ESL students has been well-documented. Therefore, ESL class participants may be at a distinct disadvantage, requiring much more time to complete course requirements than other students. We are acutely aware of not disadvantaging these participants, and consider ways of teaching/learning (e.g., role play, demonstrations, and small-group activities) that may be more helpful to them. However, we still have concerns about this situation, which is very difficult to measure or obtain accurate information about. Paraprofessionals are often the first point of contact for breastfeeding families, and can have a large impact on a family's breastfeeding experience. It essential we meet their learning needs effectively.

Additionally, other course materials (e.g., PowerPoint presentations and handouts) are written at a reading level that may be higher than what some participants can read. Targeting these materials at the appropriate reading level is difficult, as professionals expect a higher level reading and come to the class with previous college-level education and professional experiences. In practice, we have found that one size does not fit all very well.

Recently, greater emphasis has been placed on improving health care for breastfeeding families (U.S. Department of Health and Human Services, 2011). Health care agencies are insisting that providers have lactation specific education, as evidenced by the WIC and Indian Health Service agencies that regularly send new staff to our lactation courses. Another issue we have noticed that has influenced learning outcomes is related to participants whose attendance is mandated by their employers. While many participants who are required to attend our classes do so willingly, and with a genuine interest in learning, there is always a contingent that would rather be doing anything else.

We are well aware that motivation affects learning outcomes. Our pre-/posttest survey also measures beliefs about the outcomes of breast- and formula-feeding, and attitudes toward the act of breast- and formula-feeding. We have found that beliefs for all participants do not change much from pre- to post-testing, suggesting people's beliefs are not easily changed by education. Paraprofessionals have significantly greater change in their attitudes toward breastfeeding, demonstrating the importance that lactation education may have in affecting practice through attitudinal change, which may in turn have a positive effect on practice. It also supports the importance of providing lactation education to all health care providers working with breastfeeding families. Even though a portion of the class participants were required to attend our classes, their attitudes toward breastfeeding were changed positively by their attendance.

While many governmental and non-governmental agencies providing care to breastfeeding families are aware of the increased emphasis placed on having supportive services for these families is required by regulatory and other policies, not all agencies equally have by-in to the necessary changes. Additionally, in some agencies, there is a desire to improve lactation services, but little understanding of how to do it. We have seen evidence of this in the survey responses related to agency infrastructure supporting their efforts to change practice and provide evidence-based care. The Baby-Friendly Hospital Initiative provides a road map for hospitals, but there is no similar guidance for community-based agencies. Paraprofessionals, who are at the bottom of the power structure within an agency, may be the best barometer of how well an organization has operationalized practice to support and promote breastfeeding. A greater emphasis needs to be placed on understanding these dynamics.

Our findings and experiences raise a number of questions about the need for the development and use of more nuanced educational outcomes, if effective change is to occur. Perhaps conducting classes for either professionals or paraprofessional would better serve the goal of changing practice, as the specific skills needed to address the differences in the perceived (or actual) agency and position within the work environment power structures could be addressed. Knowledge is a necessary component of practice change. However, it is not sufficient to realize widespread use of best practices or to achieve national public health goals.

References

Bernaix, L. W., Schmidt, C. A., Arrizola, M., Iovinelli, D., & Medina-Poelinez, C. (2008). Success of a lactation education program on NICU nurses' knowledge and attitudes. *Journal of Obstetric, Gynecologic, & Neonatal Nursing, 37*(4), 436-445.

Chezem, J. C., Friesen, C. A., & Parker, C. G. (2004). Effect of professional postpartum support on infant feeding patterns among breastfeeding participants in the WIC program. *Family and Consumer Sciences Research Journal, 32*(4), 349-360.

Chin, A. C., Myers, L., & Magnus, J.H. (2008). Race, education, and breastfeeding initiation in Louisiana, 2000-2004. *Journal of Human Lactation, 24*(2), 175-185.

Criscco-Lizza, R. (2006). Black non-hispanic mothers' perceptions about the promotion of infant-feeding methods by nurses and physicians *JOGNN, 35*(2), 173-180.

Curley, C. M., & Li, R. (2003). Culture and ethnicity key considerations for increasing breastfeeding rates. *Journal of Human Lactation, 19*(1), 21-23.

Declercq, E., Labbok, M. H., Sakala, C., & O'Hara, M. (2009). Hospital practices and women's likelihood of fulfilling their intention to exclusively breastfeed. *American Journal of Public Health, 99*(5), 929-935.

DiGirolamo, A. M., Grummer-Strawn, L. M., & Fein, S. B. (2008). Effect of maternity-care practices on breastfeeding. *Pediatrics, 122*(Supp 2), S43-49.

Ford, C. L., & Airhihenbuwa, C. O. (2010). Critical race theory, race equity, and public health: toward antiracism praxis. *American Journal of Public Health, 100*(S1), S30-S35.

Grzywacz, J. G., McMahan, S., Hurley, J. R., Stokols, D., & Phillips, K. (2004). Serving racial and ethnic populations with health promotion. *American Journal of Health Promotion, 18*(5), 8-12.

Hillenbrand, K. M., & Larsen, P. G. (2002). Effect of an educational intervention about breastfeeding on the knowledge of confidence, and behaviors of pediatric resident physicians. *Pediatrics, 110*(5), 59-66.

Ingram, J. (2006). Multiprofessional training for breastfeeding management in primary care in the UK. *International Breastfeeding Journal, 1*(1), 9.

Ogburn, T., Espey, E., Leeman, L., & Alvarez, K. (2005). A breastfeeding curriculum for residents and medical students: A multidisciplinary approach. *Journal of Human Lactation, 21*(4), 458-464.

Renfrew, M. J., McFadden, A., Dykes, F., et al. (2006). Addressing the learning deficit in breastfeeding: strategies for change. *Maternal & Child Nutrition, 2*(4), 239-244.

Smale, M., Renfrew, M. J., Marshall, J. L., & Spiby, H. (2006). Turning policy into practice: More difficult than it seems. The case of breastfeeding education. *Maternal & Child Nutrition, 2*(2), 103-113.

U.S. Department of Health and Human Services. (2011). *The Surgeon General's call to action to support breastfeeding.* Washington, DC: U.S. Department of Health and Human Services.

Exploring Long-Term Breastfeeding in African American Women Using Positive Deviance: Implications for Research and Practice

Tyra Gross

Introduction

For decades, African Americans have the lowest breastfeeding rates in comparison to other racial groups in the United States (U.S. Department of Health and Human Services, 2010). The majority of research on breastfeeding in African American women is quantitative studies using larger data sets. Few studies have examined breastfeeding from the perspective of the African American mother (Spencer & Grassley, 2013). Qualitative methods are useful for gaining an in-depth understanding of a phenomenon and describing people's personal experiences.

Additionally, collaborative research methodologies, such as positive deviance, offer a unique approach to conducting breastfeeding research in the African American population by engaging the community throughout the research process. Over the past few decades, public health has increased efforts to promote breastfeeding among African American women. Despite rising breastfeeding rates in this population, few research studies have analyzed existing community solutions to address breastfeeding in African American women.

Positive Deviance (PD) is an asset-based problem-solving approach to community health, which aims to identify uncommon health behaviors that improve health in low-resource communities (Sternin, 2002). Very few studies have used Positive Deviance to understand breastfeeding behaviors in mothers from disenfranchised backgrounds. Ma and Magnus, (2011) published the only study to date using Positive Deviance to explore breastfeeding in African American women. In this secondary data analysis project on WIC mothers, the researchers concluded that qualitative research methods are important to examine characteristics of African American women who are positive deviants for breastfeeding.

Highlighting the personal experiences of African American women who have breastfed longer-term would fill a gap in the breastfeeding literature. This research focused on using the Positive Deviance Approach to explore the breastfeeding experiences of African American women participating in the Georgia WIC program. The purpose of the study was to understand African American women's breastfeeding experiences and to explore the factors influencing their decision to initiate and sustain breastfeeding. Specifically, 1) How did mothers form the intention to breastfeed during pregnancy, 2) What enabled mothers to initiate and sustain breastfeeding during the first few weeks after birth, and 3) What enabled mothers to continue breastfeeding for 6 months or longer? The theory of planned behavior served as the conceptual framework for this project, and guided questioning and data analysis.

Method

The methodology for this research was based on the steps of the Positive Deviance Approach (Sternin, 2002). Step 1 is defining the problem, perceived causes, and community norms. Three focus groups were held with a total of 23 Georgia WIC breastfeeding peer counselors to better define breastfeeding norms in local African American women, and understand the perceived barriers and facilitators of breastfeeding for their clients. Findings from the focus group helped the researcher refine questions for the interview phase of the study.

Step 2 is identifying individuals in the community who already exhibit the desired behavior. WIC peer counselors helped recruit participants, positive deviants, for individual interviews. To be considered positive deviants and eligible for an interview, women had to identify as African-American, currently participate in Georgia WIC, have a history breastfeeding 6 months or longer, and recently breastfed a child age 2 years or younger. Interviews were audio-recorded and professionally transcribed and analyzed using thematic analysis. Step 3 is discovering the unique practices/behaviors that enable the Positive Deviants to find better solutions to the problem than others in the community. Individual interviews were conducted with 11 African American mothers from the WIC program that had breastfed for 6 months or longer. One-hour semi-structured interviews were held either in participants' homes or another comfortable setting of the participant's choice (i.e., library, coffee shop).

Thematic analysis was used to analyze the data. Braun and Clarke (2006, p.79) state that "thematic analysis is a method for identifying, analyzing, and reporting patterns (themes) within data. It minimally organizes and describes your data set in (rich) detail." The six steps that Braun and Clark give for thematic analysis include the following: 1) Familiarizing yourself with your data, 2) Generating initial codes, 3) Searching for themes, 4) Reviewing themes, 5) Defining and naming theme, and 6) Producing the report. To familiarize myself with the data, I listened to each interview recording multiple times generated notes, and reviewed transcripts and field notes from each interview. I created a data matrix to look at which patterns were mentioned by which participants (i.e., pumping, co-sleeping, work accommodations). Using the first few transcripts and findings from the focus groups, I developed codes to use in analyzing transcripts. First, coding was done by hand by printing transcripts and writing codes in the margins. Next, quotes from each participant were compiled by codes to build themes. Themes were defined and named using constructs of the Theory of Planned Behavior as a guide.

Findings

In the sample of 11 women, ages ranged from 23 to 35 years. Women had three children on average, with 55% married and 36% having completed college degrees. In response to the first research question, patterns include WIC was a more reliable source for prenatal breastfeeding education and support than health care providers. The majority of the participants had a family history of breastfeeding. If it wasn't a mother or grandmother, it was a sister or aunt. Breastfeeding decisions did not always occur during pregnancy for the first child, and occasionally occurred shortly after birth. Breastfeeding confidence during first pregnancy was low until babies latched for the first time after birth. Just as each child is different, breastfeeding experiences differed with each child.

Regarding research question 2, mothers described that early breastfeeding support in the hospital and at home from WIC peer counselors improves mothers' breastfeeding confidence. Pumping was a common practice necessary to continue breastfeeding after women and their infants transitioned home from the hospital. Public breastfeeding was described as challenging and uncomfortable. Several participants described breastfeeding or expressing milk in public restrooms, or the backseat of their car when in public. Only one participant mentioned ever attending a support group. Lastly, patterns answering the third research question were that social support, along with staying at home, and work and school accommodations enable long-term breastfeeding. Of those reporting working or attending school, about half described adequate breastfeeding accommodations. WIC peer counselors were reliable sources of support. By 6 months postpartum, mothers have an established breastfeeding routine and are able to give infants other foods. However, maternal determination and sacrifice are personality traits required for breastfeeding success. After describing their breast-feeding experiences, participants concluded with advice for other African American mothers, health providers, and their communities on how to better support breastfeeding mothers.

Conclusion

The analysis for this research is still ongoing. However, preliminary findings highlight implications for practice, research, and policy. Additionally, preliminary findings emphasize that positive deviance can be used as a participatory research method to design culturally appropriate community breastfeeding programs and policies in support of breastfeeding African American women.

References

Braun, V., & Clarke, V. (2006). Using thematic analysis in psychology. *Qualitative Research in Psychology, 3*(2), 77-101.

Ma, P, & Magnus, J. (2011). Exploring the concept of positive deviance related to breastfeeding initiation in black and white WIC enrolled first time mothers. *Maternal and Child Health Journal, 16*(8), 1583-1593.

Spencer, B., & Grassley, J. (2013). African American women and breastfeeding: An integrative literature review. *Health Care for Women International, 34*(7), 607-625.

Sternin, J. (2002). Positive deviance: A new paradigm for addressing today's problems today. *Journal of Corporate Citizenship*, 5, 57-62.

U.S. Department of Health and Human Services. (2010). *National Immunization Survey 2007.* Retrieved from http://www.cdc.gov/breastfeeding/data/NIS_data/2007/socio-demographic_any.htm

Breastfeeding Cessation: Associations with Maternal and Infant Characteristics among African American, First-Time Mothers

Laura E. Downey, Eric A. Hodges, Amanda L. Thompson,
and Margaret E. Bentley

Overview

The American Academy of Pediatrics (AAP) recommends that women breastfeed their infants exclusively for the first 6 months, then continue breastfeeding with the addition of complementary foods until at least 12 months of age (American Academy of Pediatrics Section on Breastfeeding, 2012). The World Health Organization (WHO) extends this recommendation until at least 2 years of age (World Health Organization, 2011). Significant numbers of mothers do not meet these recommendations. Disparities exist among racial and socioeconomic groups, with non-Hispanic Black breastfeeding rates much lower than non-Hispanic Whites or Hispanics (Centers for Disease Control, 2013).

The aim of this study was to characterize maternal rationale for breastfeeding cessation among first-time, African American, WIC-eligible mothers in North Carolina, and to explore the associations of maternal depression and infant temperament with breastfeeding cessation from early infancy into toddlerhood.

Method

This study was a secondary data analysis from a primary study of African American mothers and infants, the Infant Care, Feeding, and Risk of Obesity Study (Slining et al., 2010; Thompson & Bentley, 2012; Thompson et al., 2009; Wasser et al., 2011). The design was cross-sectional, using self-report questionnaires at 3, 6, 9, 12, and 18 months postpartum to characterize WIC-eligible mothers' rationale for breastfeeding cessation, and to explore how maternal and infant characteristics were associated with breastfeeding cessation.

Inclusion criteria included being a first-time mother, 18 to 35 years of age, who was willing to participate in home visits and assessments, and who was WIC eligible (gross income at or below 185 percent of the U.S. Poverty Income Guidelines) (U.S. Department of Agriculture, 2008). Infants needed to be healthy singletons, greater than 35 weeks gestation. Exclusion criteria included any condition that might affect feeding or growth.

After the preliminary analysis between those who never breastfed and those who did, the following participants were excluded from the original sample of 217 participants: 1) mothers who never breastfed their infants, or breastfed their infants for less than one day, 2) mothers for whom breastfeeding cessation reasons were missing, or were not available in narrative form, and 3) mothers whose reported time of cessation was inconsistent across data collection visits. There were a total of 128 mother-infant dyads included in the final sample.

Mothers' reasons for breastfeeding cessation were reviewed by two coders and assigned one of 15 codes. Maternal depression was analyzed using a total Center for Epidemiological Studies-Depression (CES-D) scale. A dichotomous variable was created using the cut-off score of ≥ 16, which indicates the individual has depressive symptoms warranting further evaluation for a diagnosis of depression (Huba et al., 1995). Infant temperament was evaluated using six subscales from the- Infant Behavior Questionnaire-Revised (IBQ-R) at 3, 6, and 9 months. Toddler temperament was evaluated using five subscales from the Early Childhood Behavior Questionnaire (ECBQ) at 12 and 18 months.

Statistical Analysis

Chi-square tests were conducted to ascertain whether maternal depression and sociodemographic variables were significantly associated with mothers having ever breastfed. Associations among breastfeeding status and maternal age were explored with t-tests.

Among the subsample of 128 mother-infant dyads who had ever engaged in breastfeeding, the relationships of both intended and actual duration of breastfeeding with sociodemographic variables, reasons for breastfeeding cessation, depressive symptoms in mothers, and infant temperament were explored at each time point with X^2 or Fisher's Exact Test, correlations, and independent samples t-tests, as appropriate. Descriptive statistics were assessed for all variables.

A series of binary logistic regression models for breastfeeding cessation were modeled at 3 months due to the small number of those continuing to breastfeed beyond 3 months. Statistically significant demographic covariates and maternal depression (dichotomized by a score of $<$ or $\geq$ 16 on the CES-D) were included in each model. Subsequent models included single dimensions of temperament that were found to be significantly associated with maternal depression at 3 months.

Results

In the preliminary analysis of the full sample of 217 Infant Care Study participants, mothers with less education were less likely to have ever breastfed. Slightly less than a quarter (22.8%) of mothers who ever breastfed had less than a high school education, while 40% of mothers who never breastfed had achieved a less than high school education, X^2 (1) = 6.41, $p<0.05$. Slightly less than half (47.8%) of mothers who ever breastfed had achieved a less than college education, while 76.9% of mothers who never breastfed had a less than college education, X^2 (1) = 15.24, $p<0.001$.

The average duration of breastfeeding for participants was 3.09 ± 3.85 months (N= 125). Mothers who stopped breastfeeding by 6 months (n = 15) had a significantly shorter mean intended duration of breastfeeding compared to those who breastfed beyond 6 months (n = 18) (6.40 ± 1.92 months versus 8.83 ± 2.91 months; t (29.57) = -2.87, p = .007).

Qualitative data suggested that women often discontinued breastfeeding due to perceived insufficient supply, disruption, work, biting, and self-weaning of their infants. Many of these issues were amenable to intervention. Mothers who cited insufficient supply and pain as reasons for cessation were significantly more likely to stop breastfeeding by 3 months than those who continued breastfeeding. Among mothers who stopped breastfeeding by 3 months, 44.1% cited insufficient supply as the reason for cessation compared to 21.9% of mothers feeding beyond 3 months, X^2 (1) = 4.97, p = .03. 12.9% of mothers stopping by 3 months cited pain as the reason for cessation compared to 0% of mothers feeding beyond 3 months, Fisher's Exact Test, p = .036.

Maternal education was significantly associated with breast-feeding cessation at 3 months. Slightly more than half (53.4%) of mothers who stopped breastfeeding at 3 months had achieved a high school or less, while 74.3% of mothers breastfeeding beyond 3 months had some college or higher-level education, X^2 (1) = 7.74, p = .005.

Maternal age and single marital status were significantly associated with breastfeeding cessation at 3 months. Over three quarters (78.2%) of unmarried mothers (combination of never married and separated) stopped breastfeeding by 3 months compared to 38.9% of married mothers, Fisher's Exact test, $p = .001$. Mothers who stopped breastfeeding by 3 months were significantly younger (22.44 ± 3.44 years) than mothers who fed beyond 3 months (24.49 ± 4.45 years), t (123) = 2.75, $p = .007$. However, married mothers ($n = 18$) were significantly older (26.98 ± 4.52 years) compared to unmarried mothers ($n = 107$) (22.35 ± 3.30 years), t (20.16) = 4.16, $p \le .001$.

Depression was significantly associated with breastfeeding cessation at 3 months. Mothers who stopped breastfeeding by 3 months had significantly higher mean scores on the CES-D compared to mothers who fed beyond 3 months, t (109.14) = 3.65, $p < .001$. Thirty-three percent of the mothers who stopped breastfeeding by 3 months had CES-D depression scores ≥16 compared to only 8.6% of mothers who breastfed beyond 3 months, X^2 (1) = 7.74, $p = .005$.

Infant temperament was significantly associated with breastfeeding cessation at 9 months. Mothers who stopped breastfeeding by 9 months reported significantly higher scores on the *Duration of Orienting* temperament subscale on IBQ-R compared to those mothers who continued breastfeeding beyond 9 months, t (16) = 2.46, $p = 0.03$). Mothers who stopped breastfeeding by 9 months reported significantly higher scores on the *Low Intensity Pleasure* temperament subscale on the IBQ-R compared to those mothers who continued breastfeeding beyond 9 months, t (16) = 2.60, $p = 0.02$).

Mothers with depressive symptoms warranting further evaluation (CES-D scores ≥ 16) were four times as likely to discontinue breastfeeding by 3 months compared to those with lower levels of depressive symptoms (Model 1). The addition of *Activity Level, Distress to Limitations*, or *Duration of Orienting* (Models 2-4) did not lead to statistically significantly improvement over Model 1 with depression alone, nor were these temperament dimensions significantly associated with breastfeeding cessation. However, the addition of any of these temperament dimensions did improve the correct classification of mothers who stopped breastfeeding by 3 months or continued beyond.

Conclusions

Our findings that mothers in this study were most likely to stop breastfeeding around 3 months indicate that interventions should target the first 3 months of life. Given associations between intended duration of breastfeeding and actual duration of breastfeeding, it is particularly important to discuss breastfeeding prenatally. The statistically significant reasons cited for breastfeeding cessation by 3 months, insufficient supply and pain, are both amenable to intervention. Given the association between higher depression scores and breastfeeding cessation, along with infant temperament associations with maternal depression, there is a need for improved screening and treatment of postpartum depression. Findings related to maternal depression and infant temperament represent important areas for future research in breastfeeding support.

References

American Academy of Pediatrics, Section on Breastfeeding. (2012). Breastfeeding and the use of human milk. *Pediatrics, 129*(3), e827-e841.

Centers for Disease Control and Prevention (CDC). (2013). Progress in increasing breastfeeding and reducing racial/ethnic differences — United States, 2000–2008 Births, *Morbidity and Mortality Weekly Report (MMWR), 62*(5), 77.

Huba, G. J., Melchior, L. A., Staff at the Measurement Group, & HRSA/HAB's SPNS Cooperative Agreement Steering Committee. (1995). Module 26A: CES-D Form [Interview]. *Culver City, California: The Measurement Group,* [Online].

Slining, M., Adair, L. S., Goldman, B. D., Borja, J. B., & Bentley, M. (2010). Infant overweight is associated with delayed motor development. *The Journal of pediatrics,157*(1), 20-25.

Thompson, A. L., & Bentley, M. E. (2012). The critical period of infant feeding for the development of early disparities in obesity. *Social science & medicine (1982)*.

Thompson, A. L., Mendez, M. A., Borja, J. B., Adair, L. S., Zimmer, C. R., & Bentley, M. E. (2009), Development and validation of the Infant Feeding Style Questionnaire. *Appetite, 53*(2), 210-221.

U.S. Department of Agriculture (USDA). (2008). *Income Eligibility Guidelines 2008-2009, 73*(68).

Wasser, H., Bentley, M., Borja, J., Davis Goldman, B., Thompson, A., Slining, M., & Adair, L. (2011). Infants perceived as "fussy" are more likely to receive complementary foods before 4 months. *Pediatrics, 127*(2), 229-237.

World Health Organization (WHO). (2011, January 15)., *Exclusive breastfeeding for six months best for babies everywhere*. Available: http://www.who.int/mediacentre/news/statements/2011/breastfeeding_20110115/en/ [2013, 01/10].

Infant Feeding Practices among Somali-born Women Who Have Migrated to Bristol, UK

Susan Young

Abstract

In recent years, Bristol has provided refuge to many women who fled the conflict in Somalia. The study presented here focuses on the infant feeding practices, primarily breastfeeding, of a group of Somali-born women living in the city. Framed by an anthropological perspective, the study seeks to understand breastfeeding within the wider contexts of the women's lives and their experiences of transition from one country to another. Concepts of transnationalism contribute to the theorizing and methodological approach. A hallmark of any migrant group is the triadic relationship between their homeland, their collectively identified ethnic group in the place of arrival, and the existing sociocultural contexts where the group now resides. Therefore, information has been gathered from these three dimensions: Somali homeland breastfeeding practices, the Bristol context for breastfeeding as represented by health care services, and the current infant feeding practices of a group of immigrant Somali-born women. Since Somalia is closed to travellers, information about homeland breastfeeding practices relies on accounts from older women, and a handful of written sources. The core of the study is a small ethnography carried out during one year with mothers who have children under the age of 3 who attended a family-center play session.

I talked with the mothers not only about infant-feeding practices, but also conversed informally about a wide range of topics in order to gain insight in to their wider beliefs and experiences. The study includes semi-structured interviews with 11 professionals employed as midwives and health visitors who work in majority Somali areas in UK cities. The interpretation formulates the different versions of breastfeeding beliefs and practices revealed by the three dimensions of the study, and considers the relationships between them. I argue that consideration of the women's multiple positions from a transnational perspective helps to explain their breastfeeding practices.

Background and Aims

This ongoing study explores the infant feeding practices of Somali-born women now living in Bristol (a city in South West England), who arrived as refugees escaping the Somali civil war. Since almost without exception, Somali women breastfeed their babies, breastfeeding is the central focus of the study. Taking an anthropological perspective, I have observed, enquired about, and documented the women's practices with an aim to understand how these practices are woven into the wider sociocultural contexts of their lives. However, as a consequence of migration, their circumstances have profoundly and rapidly changed. This is particularly true for women arriving from pre-industrial, Islamic Somalia to the post-industrial, mainly secular UK. This draws attention to the process through which a legacy of practices from their homeland—either directly experienced, remembered, or told to them by elders—becomes transformed through the experiences of migration.

Identifying the homeland traditions, the post-migration changes and the factors implicated in change, may appear to be relatively straightforward tasks. However, a fundamental argument framing this study is that ethnocentric concepts lie behind constructs of infant feeding both in academia and professional practice. Around breastfeeding, a certain ideological concept of mothering that is exclusive and based on attachment within a small heterosexual family unit dominates much of Western thinking. These constructs of infant feeding privilege certain concepts and neglect alternatives, such as the cooperative nature of infant care by larger kinship groups and communities, Islamic meanings attached to breastfeeding, differently defined gender roles and relationships, and infant feeding priorities where infant mortality rates are high. Anthropologists have contributed a range of rich and diverse accounts of infant feeding from differing cultural circumstances that take account of the culturally variable social structures in which infant feeding takes place and the meanings granted to breastfeeding (e.g., Mabilia, 2005; Maher, 1992; Van Esterik, 2012). However, in my view, these ideas remain marginal to mainstream discourses around breastfeeding.

Theoretical Perspective

There is well-placed concern among health professionals to support the infant feeding of migrant women who have settled in the mainly English speaking and affluent countries of the North (see Schmied et al., 2012). This concern has led to a number of studies that document their infant feeding, often with comparisons to resident populations. Driven by public-health agendas, these studies typically arrive at suggestions for interculturally sensitive health-service practice based on lists of cultural characteristics. While these studies document "traditional" practices, and then describe what has changed or continued, often assuming change to be a linear acculturation from homeland to host-land practices, they rarely explore the process of change, nor propose a way to theorize it.

Reading contemporary literature around migration suggests some possible ways to theorize the process of change. In recent years, a significant shift in thinking around migration has occurred as a consequence of increased mobility, new technologies of communication and money transfer systems. Individuals are no longer understood as necessarily tied to where they reside, but may maintain active ties to two or more locations and sustain multiple allegiances, referred to as transnationalism (Vertovec, 2009). Thus, the Somali women I spoke with had, between them, family members in Finland, the Netherlands, Canada, Somalia, Somaliland, and Kenya, as well as religious callings to the Middle East. Several spoke daily with family members in other countries. Transnationalism offers theoretical frameworks that are not based on acculturation or multiculturalism, but on more flexible and varying models of adaptation. Nederveen-Pieterse's (2010) notion of flexible acculturation is, in my view, one of the most useful because it emphasises complex interplays and dialogues between differences. Importantly, it also acknowledges both individual agency, and the constraints and possibilities afforded by the social, cultural, and political environment.

Method

Over the course of one year, I participated in a mother and under-3s group serving an area of majority Somali population in inner-city Bristol. Here, I could talk with and observe a group of Somali-born mothers with babies and very young children. There were five regular attenders, and several others who attended intermittently. The mothers knew that I was interested in infant feeding and would volunteer information or respond to questions. I also joined in wider ranging, informal conversations that gave me information and insights in to the wider circumstances of their everyday lives. Towards the end of the year, I carried out some semi-structured interviews with four of the mothers and a Somali worker, herself a mother. In addition, I have interviewed 11 breastfeeding-support professionals working in Somali-majority areas. Two were Somali-born mothers who talked about both their personal experiences of feeding, and those of the women they supported.

The field notes and interview data have been analysed to arrive at a number of core themes.

Some Initial Interpretations

The study brings together the homeland practices as identified from literature and remembered accounts: infant feeding in the host country as identified by the professional, policy-informed model, and the observations and accounts provided by the Somali-born women participating in the study. Somali infant-feeding practices, like those of any group, developed over time in a specific geographical, historical, cultural, social, and economic environment, albeit varied by income, clan, and location (urban or rural). However, there are some strong unifying factors: the Islamic faith; the close-knit extended family and neighborhood communities providing support and actively contributing to the raising of children; the colonial background; the harshness of the environment; food insecurities and poor health provision leading to malnutrition and high rates of infant mortality. As a country based largely on nomadic herding of goats, sheep, cows, and camels, milk plays a central role as not only a primary source of nutrition but also, particularly with camel milk, of symbolic importance in Somali identity.

Motherhood has high status in Somali society, and the birth of a baby is a "special time," as explained to me, for the mother. Breastfeeding is the norm and is widely encouraged by both family and Islam. However, mixed feeding is also a norm, and all the mothers I interviewed supplemented with formula milk. Far from being an acquired practice on arrival in the UK, as assumed by the breastfeeding professionals, formula milk merely replaces the animal milks and water that have always been given to Somali infants. The tendency for Somali women, according to health professionals, to 'overfeed" their babies, resulting in weight gains at the top of measurement scales, has been noticed (e.g., Steinman et al., 2010). Peer and family pressure to have plump babies was intense, as I observed and was told. When I asked why, the mothers reported that plump babies look beautiful and are healthy.

Following arrival in Bristol, all the mothers referred to the difficulties of "being on their own," and the loss of the extended family and social network. They spoke of frequently "not knowing what to do" in relation to infant care, and told of phoning relatives in other countries for basic information and advice. Many women have large families and close birth spacing. In Somalia, children aged 3 or 4 years would be outside playing with other children, and care would be shared with older relatives, leaving the mothers to focus on care of the very youngest. Large families persist as an ideal, post-migration, yet lacking help, in poorly equipped and over-crowded social housing, the women often struggle to manage.

Male partners, in contrast to the Western assumptions of marriage as the primary close bond in a nuclear family, play a more marginal role. It is not uncommon in Bristol for women to live on their own with small children, either because their husband remains in Somalia, is displaced, has elected to live elsewhere, has a second partner, or is divorced. However, while migration may have heightened the instability of marriage, this is not a recent characteristic of family structure (Lewis, 1994).

Several have discussed the role that the Islamic religion increasingly plays in migrant Somali life, and how it offers security, self-esteem, and solace (see Griffiths, 2002; Harris, 2004). Some women quoted Islamic doctrine for infants to be breastfed for 2 years as an ideal to aspire to. The religious dimension, from what they said, appeared to be bound with obligation and duty to others. Two women talking together said that they were making a special connection with their babies by giving them their own milk. While cautious of over-interpreting from scant data, in dominant Western constructs of breastfeeding, the socioemotional value of breastfeeding is assumed to lie in psychological concepts of attachment, of prime future benefit to the baby, whereas the legacy of Islamic beliefs around milk kinship may locate the socioemotional value in cementing relational ties of future benefit to the mother.

Conclusion

In considering how infant feeding practices transform post-migration, and adopting flexible acculturation as a theoretical frame, it appears that some practices shift easily, and are susceptible or amenable to influence while others are more persistent. This may relate to surface and deep-seated elements of childrearing, mothering, and infant-feeding culture. The surface elements may be flexible, while the deeper attitudes, values, and beliefs, forming a structural ensemble, a kind of cultural grammar, remain more immutable. Drawing on evidence so far, their infant feeding practices seem to crystallize in to a "best fit in the circumstances," adaptive model. The surface-level flexibility is driven by pragmatism and strategic decision-making that attempts to balance the mothers,' family members,' and infants' best interests within structural constraints imposed by poor housing, low income, and institutional health provision.

References

Griffiths, D. J. (2002). *Somali and Kurdish refugees in London: New identities in the diaspora.* Aldershot: Ashgate.

Harris, H. (2004). The Somali community in the UK: What we know and how we know it. Report commissioned by The information Centre about Asylum and Refugees in the UK (ICAR) Available from: www. icar.org.uk/somalicommunityreport.pdf *accessed 10 October 2013.*

Lewis, I. M. (1994). *Blood and bone: The call of kinship in somali society.* Lawrenceville, NJ: The Red Sea Press.

Mabilia, M. (2005). *Breast feeding and sexuality: Behaviour, beliefs and taboos among the Gogo mothers in Tanzania.* (M. S. Ash, Trans.). New York: Berghahn Books.

Maher, V. (Ed.). (1992). *The anthropology of breastfeeding: Natural law or social construct.* Oxford: Berg Publishers.

Nederveen-Pieterse, J. (2010). Global multiculturalism, flexible acculturation. *Transcience Journal, 1*(1), 87-105.

Schmied, V., Olley, H., Burns, E., Duff, M., Dennis, C-L., & Dahlen, H.G. (2012). Contradictions and conflict: A meta-ethnographic study of migrant women's experiences of breastfeeding in a new country. *BMC Pregnancy and Childbirth, 12,* 163.

Steinman, L., Doescher, M., Keppel, G. A., Pak-Gorstein, S., Graham, E., Haq, A., Johnson, D. B., & Spicer, P. (2010). Understanding infant feeding beliefs, practices and preferred nutrition education and health provider approaches: an exploratory study with Somali mothers in the USA. *Maternal and Child Nutrition, 6*(1), 67-88.

Van Esterik, P. (2012). Breastfeeding across cultures: dealing with difference. In P. Hall Smith, B. L. Hausmann, & M. Labbok, *Beyond health, beyond choice: breastfeeding constraints and realities* (pp. 53-63). New Brunswick: Rutgers University Press.

Vertovec, S. (2009). *Transnationalism.* London: Routledge.

Section IIb

LGBTQ Reproductive Health

Changing Demographic Patterns for LGBT Parent-Headed Families and Implications for Breastfeeding

W. Roger Mills-Koonce, Bharathi Zvara, Nicole Heilbron,
Hongjian Cao, and Claire Wood

As compared to opposite-sex parents, lesbian mothers and gay fathers encounter many unique and challenging experiences and decisions when it comes to starting a family with children. A recent Institute of Medicine Report (2011) concluded that "The role of parenthood in adult development among LGBT [lesbian, gay, bisexual, or transgender] people is also not well understood [...] research examining the formation and experiences of families among LGBT individuals, as well as other social influences, would contribute to a fuller understanding of LGBT health" (p. 297), and even less is known about family structure and the topic of breastfeeding within LGBT parent-headed households. For gay males, there are decisions related to adoption or various forms of surrogacy. For lesbian females, there are similar decisions about adoption, donor insemination, or in vitro fertilization.

For same-sex couples committed to maximizing the biological kinship between each parent and their offspring, great efforts are made to promote biological egalitarianism for each parent. For a gay male couple, this may involve choosing to use one partner's sperm and using the egg from a female family member of the other partner.

For a lesbian female couple, this may involve choosing to extract the egg from one partner and implanting the fertilized egg into the uterus of the other partner. These decisions may also influence the establishment and consolidation of caregiving roles and childrearing decisions, such as breastfeeding. Although many same-sex parents feel that both social and biological factors influence the connectedness between parents and offspring, and that, among lesbian couples, bonding opportunities aren't necessarily diminished as a function of one partner not breastfeeding (Goldberg, Downing, & Sauck, 2008). It is very likely that decisions about breastfeeding both influence, and are influenced by, decisions about family formation and caregiving roles in same-sex couples. Next, we provide a brief review of the issues surrounding the changing demography of same-sex, parent-headed households, and then discuss how these trends may relate to decisions about breastfeeding.

Changing Demographic Trends for LGBT Parents

The American Academy of Child & Adolescent Psychiatry (2006) estimated that there are millions of children living with LGBT parents in the United States (see also Black, Gates, Sanders, & Taylor, 2000; Gates, 2013). U.S. Census data indicate that there are same-sex, parent-headed households in more than 75% of U.S. counties, suggesting that same-sex parent-headed households are not limited to specific communities or geographic areas, but rather are represented in urban and rural communities, and both socially progressive and conservative states (Gates, 2011). Although common stereotypes of same-sex family formation include adoption for gay fathers, and sperm donation for lesbian mothers, these methods only reflect a portion of same-sex parent-headed families. Until recently, the majority of children of lesbian or gay parents were conceived from prior heterosexual unions in which parents (prior to coming out as having same-sex attractions) produced a child through sexual intercourse with someone from the opposite sex (Gates, 2008). However, this experience is becoming less common as cultural norms in the U.S. have shifted towards greater acceptance of lesbian and gay individuals, and increasing numbers of young adults openly acknowledge their same-sex attraction in advance of entering heterosexual unions. The result of this cultural shift, however, is that more lesbian and gay adults are making decisions about their methods of family formation as openly lesbian or gay individuals or couples. These decisions may have implications for the choices LGBT parents make with regard to breastfeeding.

What we currently know is that LGBT parent-headed households compromise a very heterogeneous group of families (Gates & Sell, 2006), and this heterogeneity is likely to increase with the decline of childbearing in prior opposite-sex unions for many LGBT individuals. Furthermore, the sociodemographics of LGBT families are likely to change as a function of this trend. For example, based on our best estimates from U.S. Census data and other representative samples of American families, same-sex couples with biological children (a majority of whom are from prior opposite-sex relationships) are at greater economic disadvantage, have lower education levels, are more likely to be racial/ethnic minorities, and are more likely to live in the socially more conservative Southern and Midwestern regions of the country as compared to same-sex parents with adopted children (Gates, 2011). These differences likely exist for two reasons. The first is that these same sociodemographic risk factors are associated with younger rates of childbearing, meaning that lower-income and lower-education individuals (as compared to individuals with higher incomes and higher levels of education) are likely to have children at younger ages prior to coming out as an LGBT individual.

The second reason for these sociodemographic discrepancies is that the high cost of adoption may be prohibitive for lower-income LGBT individuals. Thus, there may be two potential selection effects here at work, one in which lower-income individuals are selecting into opposite-sex childbearing early in life prior to coming out, and one in which lower-income LGBT are selected out of adoption due to the financial costs. However, as we see rates of prior opposite-sex child-bearing decline for LGBT parents, most are now left with decisions of adoption or surrogacy (for gay fathers) or donor insemination or in vitro fertilization (for lesbian mothers). Generally speaking, each of these options are costlier than biological childbearing in opposite-sex couples, and the degree to which a same-sex couple wants to promote biological kinship for each parent further increases these costs. In other words, although the diversity in family formation methods may be increasing for LGBT parents as a function of societal and techno-logical advances, the financial costs of these methods may results in a decrease in the economic diversity of LGBT parent-headed household as fewer low-income LGBT individuals will be able to have one or multiple children via adoption or alternative reproduction methods.

Implications for Breastfeeding within LGBT Parent-Headed Families

To our knowledge, there is little-to-no research examining how these demographic shifts (both in structure and in the socioeconomics) may relate to breastfeeding behaviors within LGBT parent-headed fami-lies. In the absence of empirical literature on these topics, let us first consider possible implications of demographic changes and breast-feeding decisions for lesbian mothers. For single lesbian mothers, the decisions about breastfeeding may be similar to those faced by single heterosexual mothers; however, for same-sex female couples, the decision about breastfeeding may be more complicated. As compared to opposite-sex relations, both members of the female same-sex couple (generally speaking) are capable of breastfeeding. For couples that choose to adopt a non-biological child, the couple must decide whether neither, one, or both mothers will attempt to induce lacta-tion to support breastfeeding opportunities for the child. Although the benefits of breastfeeding adopted children have been well-docu-mented (Gribble, 2006), the decisions and considerations about "if" and "who" are unique for each same-sex female couple. These decisions may be further amplified when the method of family formation involves some variation of producing a biological child. Although the mother who carries and gives birth to the child may feel a more natural inclination to breastfeed, it is quite possible that both mothers, or only the non-birth mother, will participate. Because of their biological capacities, these decisions can be made collaboratively by the couple, who themselves can determine what is best for each parent, the child, and the family unit as a whole. It is likely that factors, such as which mother most wanted to have children, the type of work and work schedules for each mother, and unique personal characteristics of each mother, will affect these decisions. From a family-demography perspective, it is possible that these decisions will be made in advance of the child's conception and may influence the choice of method of family formation. Likewise, it is also possible that the choice of family formation method may influence decisions regarding whether neither, only one, or both mothers participate in breastfeeding.

The issues surrounding breastfeeding for LGBT fathers are different, but no less complicated. Although breastfeeding may not be a viable option for children who are adopted through public or private organizations, it is possible that gay fathers may establish arrangements with surrogate mothers to breastfeed after the child has transitioned to the custody of the fathers, or alternatively donate human milk for the fathers to provide the children. This practice may also support the continued involvement of surrogates in the lives of the adoptive fathers and children, an arrangement some gay fathers have pursued to foster a relationship between children and their birth mothers (Downing, Richardson, Kinkler, & Goldberg, 2009). Of course, these decisions also may come at increased financial costs to families, and may not be feasible for those with lower incomes.

Areas of Future Research

Despite considerable interest in the functioning and welfare of LGBT parents and their children within political, judicial, and social spheres (Patterson, 2009), there remains limited empirical research on this population, and almost none on the topic of breastfeeding (for an exception, see following chapters in this volume). We do know that the demography of LGBT parent-headed households has, and will continue to, change in the foreseeable future. Changing societal attitudes towards the topics of sexuality and gender are encouraging LGBT individuals to openly acknowledge their sexual identity earlier in life. And changing attitudes towards same-sex marriage and parenthood are challenging the collective, heteronormative definitions of "family" in the United States.

LGBT individuals and couples have more options for starting families with children (although these options are often constrained by financial costs), and these increases in options also come with increases in decisions to be made regarding breastfeeding (for both LGBT female and male individuals and couples). Future research is needed to better understand the interplay between decisions on how to start a family, and how those decisions are related to breastfeeding. This information is needed for doctors and nurses, family-planning counselors, and lactation experts, all of whom should all be well-versed in these issues to provide the best guidance and support for LGBT individuals and couples as they transition to parenthood. It is important that future research on breastfeeding be more inclusive of diverse populations, such as LGBT parents, and that future studies on LGBT family processes examine breastfeeding decisions and behaviors as a component of their research.

References

American Academy of Child & Adolescent Psychiatry. (2006). *Facts for families: Children with lesbian, gay, bisexual and transgender parents.* Retrieved from http://www.aacap.org

Black, D., Gates, G. J., Sanders, S., & Taylor, L. (2000). Demographics of the gay and lesbian population in the United States: Evidence from available systematic data sources. *Demography, 37,* 139-154.

Downing, J., Richardson, H., Kinkler, L., & Goldberg, A. (2009). Making the decision: Factors influencing gay men's choice of an adoption path. *Adoption Quarterly, 12*(3-4), 247-271.

Gates, G. J. (2008). Diversity among same-sex couples and their children. In S. Coontz (Ed.), *American families: A multicultural reader,* (2nd ed.). New York: Routledge.

Gates, G. J. (2011). Family formation and raising children among same-sex couples. *National Council on Family Relations: Family Focus on LGBT Families, FF51,* 1-3.

Gates, G. J. (2013). Geography of the LGBT population. In A. K. Baumle (Ed.), *International handbook on the demography of sexuality* (pp. 229-242). Netherlands: Springer.

Gates, G. J., & Sell, R. L. (2006). Measuring gay and lesbian couples. In S. Hofferth and L. Casper (Eds.), *The handbook of measurement issues in family research.* New York: Lawrence Erlbaum Associates, Inc.

Goldberg, A. E., Downing, J. B., & Sauck, C. C. (2008). Choices, challenges, and tensions: Perspectives of lesbian prospective adoptive parents. *Adoption Quarterly, 10*(2), 33-64.

Gribble, K. D. (2006). Mental health, attachment, and breastfeeding: Implications for adopted children and their mothers. *International Breastfeeding Journal, 1*(5), 1-15.

Institute of Medicine. (2011). *The health of lesbian, gay, bisexual, and transgender people: Building a foundation for better understanding.* Washington, DC: National Academy Press.

Patterson, C. J. (2009). Children of lesbian and gay parents: Psychology, law, and policy. *American Psychologist, 64*(8), 727-736.

You, Me, and the Other: Transgender People in the Workplace

Laurel Falconi

I came across an article in the *Toronto Star* on Monday, January 20, 2014 entitled, "Transgender Man[1] Caught in Pregnancy Fight." The article depicted the story of an individual who physically transitioned from a female to a male, but was still able to carry a baby to term because he kept his female anatomy. He was denied care from Baystate Health organization in Massachusetts because he was "too masculine" to have a baby (Gerster, 2014). The institution argued that they were not properly equipped to treat transgender patients at the time, even though they claimed to be "transgender friendly." In response to the transgender man requesting care, they opened up a separate wing in the clinic for transgender people to seek help in becoming parents. According to the transman in the article, people have a hard time wrapping their minds around anything visibly different. With this in mind, I set out to explore why transgender people's identity and existence appears confusing to many. Using qualitative interviews of a transwoman and her coworkers in a workplace setting, I am investigating how people conceptualize and

---

1 Transgender people are people whose gender identity does not match the sexual organs assigned to them at birth, as opposed to cis-gendered people whose gender identity aligns itself with sex morphology (Johnson, 2013). Some, but not all, eventually transition into the sex that matches their self-identity through hormone drug therapy and/or sex reassignment surgery (Schilt & Wiswall, 2008; Turkewitz, 2012; Taranowski, 2008; Walworth, 2003).

interpret the nature of gender classification in the presence of a transgender person who provides opportunity within social interactions to perform and reinterpret gender.

Within Canadian and American society, there are norms about what it is to be male and female that guide most people's behavior and physical appearance. These categorizations are deeply embedded within the social structure that they appear natural (West & Zimmerman, 1987). As such, disrupting the "natural" expectation of one's gender can be anxiety provoking for many. Through the performances people make and the way they dress regarding their gender identities, they are categorized into male and female. The question, "what are you?" underlies every social interaction because people need to know how to interact with you based on whether you are male or female.

The workplace provides a rich opportunity to assess these social processes, as it is an important site in which identities are enabled, negotiated, and constrained (Hines, 2010). People who are struggling with their gender identity face greater challenges in the workplace because the division of labor reinforces patterns of dominance and submission (Lester, 2008). There is a full body of literature examining workplace experiences expressing several positive and negative reactions with regard to what is classified as normal according to gender. These classifications may be done covertly, as most people are hesitant to openly express their fears, concerns, and judgments (Bonilla-Silva, 2006), since it is not condoned in a work environment. Nonetheless, it does not refute the existence of these feelings.

Coworkers are an important part of the workplace experience with transgender people because they interact with each other every day. However, in much of the literature, coworkers' points of views are not explored directly (Schilt & Connell, 2007). Understanding how people perceive gender performance addresses gender inequalities, including hidden privileges that are found not only for one's gender, but also for race, class, and other socially dominant groups. Drawing on Bonilla-Silva's (2006) concept of "color-blind racism," I argue that transgender people in the workplace bring gender to the forefront of interaction, and it influences the gender expectations, experiences, and behaviors of employee's social interactions.

In order explore these ideas, I carried out qualitative interviews at an Information Technology (IT) sector at a workplace in Canada. Over the course of several months, I interviewed a transwoman who recently underwent hormone therapy and surgery while remaining at the same workplace, as well as 10 of her coworkers (eight self-identified as female and two self- identified as male). They were all highly educated developers, analysts, or supervisors/managers. Pseudonyms are used to protect their identities.

My preliminary analysis of the transcripts has, so far highlighted performing gender in the workplace related to West and Zimmerman (1987) and Judith Butler's work on "doing gender," as well as the concept of cis-privilege and color- (or in this case, gender-) blind racism inspired by Bonilla-Silva (2006).

Gender as a Binary

The initial finding regarding gender reproduction emphasizes actions that adhere to the ideologies that gender is a binary (Johnson, 2013). Although participants may not agree with the concept, many are aware that gender is embedded as "either/or" in society. Referring to a neighbor, Mindy, a senior credit analyst believed that there are male-oriented jobs, such as mowing the lawn, and female jobs, such as planting flowers, despite the fact that men and women may do both.

A Gendered Performance

Gender as a binary underlies various social interactions, so some transgender people themselves may try to overdo their gender performances to fit in with expectations (Garfinkel, 1967). When asked if Caroline, the transwoman, did so, Mindy replied, "She, well, I think, well, she is very conscientious about her appearance, but in a conservative way, in a very office appropriate way." Kelly, a manager in the IT department stated, "FEMININE. Absolutely, feminine from the get-go, but I think Caroline was trying, from the very beginning, maybe trying too hard to fit that feminine role." She also explained that Caroline has been working on her voice for a long time now, trying to get it to that "female tone." Li, another IT supervisor, explained that, "She probably has a model or [in her] imagination says, like, 'females should behave that way,' like the body language was weird, like today it's much better; it's more normal." There appeared to be a general agreement that Caroline held to very traditional gender roles in the way she carried herself, but they seemed unnatural because she was overemphasizing expectations of being a passive, delicate female.

Coworkers' Behavior

Many participants felt that they were policing their own behaviors, in addition to Caroline's behavior. Frank shared a number of ways in which he felt "very, very self-conscious of [his] actions and pronouns around her." He admitted that he was always tempted to "hit [Caroline] on the back" as he typically did with male coworkers, but realized it was not acceptable behavior with a woman, and feared being called out by HR.

Not only did people become self-conscious about how they treated her, but also about what her appearance and actions said about their own. Some of the female participants noted that they were shocked at how good she looked, and began to look at their own clothes, accessories, and hairstyles. Jackie, a quality assurance test analyst, laughed about how she doesn't wear much jewelry and likes sports, which she realized is not considered feminine. Claire noted how Caroline used to hold doors open for people, but no longer does because she may think that as a woman, it is not expected of her. West and Zimmerman (1987) note that we can never avoid doing gender, even if we are not conscious of it, because interactions are constantly gendered, whether it is salient or not.

Cis-Privilege and Gender-Blindness

Building on Bonilla-Silva's (2006) idea about color-blind racism, the extent to which blindness to gender reinforces cis-privilege is evident when analyzing gender relations at this workplace. Employees maintained that gender and homophobia at work is no longer an issue. When asked about gender and work, Ronald stated that he thought gendering in the workplace is still there but "just not as predominant as way back when." Additionally, others emphasized the idea that gender should not matter because work should be about whoever is the most qualified. A number of other coworkers stated that Caroline plays the "transgender card," which was akin to Bonilla-Silva's (2006) explanation of the "race-card," that Caucasians argue African Americans use, in order to justify discriminatory thoughts and behaviors by placing responsibility on the "other."

Almost all of the participants spoke in terms of other people: "Others think that..." avoiding "I" so as not to incriminate themselves because they felt they did not have the same protection that Caroline had with regard to protection against discrimination in the workplace. As one respondent, Jackie, put it, "They sort of started off by telling, by saying, like, and reminding people that Caroline was protected under the law. It sort of puts people's backs up." She and others maintained that it might have been best for Caroline if she started at a new company.

The concern for the other person may harken to similar patterns, discussed by Bonilla-Silva (2006) in terms of "white flight" when "too many" people of color begin moving into white neighborhoods. His respondents noted that the shifting racial composition of neighborhoods had nothing to do with whites wanting to leave, but that perhaps members of the minority group wanted to be grouped together (Bonilla-Silva, 2006). Similarly, many of Caroline's coworkers seemed to take a paternalistic "for her own good" idea, in that perhaps it would have been better if she began working somewhere else, where her previous identity as a man was unknown. Despite these feelings, some participants did say that Caroline opened their eyes to others' gendered behaviors, including family members.

From these narratives so far, we can deduce that people are generally uncomfortable with change, and uneasy about their negative feelings toward this change. Discrepancy between how people really feel, and what they think they are expected to feel makes it difficult for them to accept more complexities of people's identities. Caroline noted, "It is also a transition for my coworkers, not just me," reiterating that gender is a relational, and complex aspect of human relations that move beyond a black and white depiction of being male or female.

References

Bonilla-Silva, E. (2006). *Racism without racists: Color-blind racism and the persistence of racial inequality in the United States.* Lanham, MD Rowman & Littlefield Publishers.

Garfinkel, H. (1967). *Studies in ethnomethodology.* Englewood Cliffs, NJ: Prentice-Hall.

Gerster, J. (2014). Transgendered man caught in pregnancy fight. *The Toronto Star, Jan 20.*

Hines, S. (2010). Queerly situated? Exploring negotiations of trans queer subjectivities at work and within community spaces in the UK. *Gender, Place, and Culture, 17*(5), 597-613.

Johnson, J. R. (2013). Cisgender privilege, intersectionality, and the criminalization of CeCe McDonald: Why intercultural communication needs transgender studies. *Journal of International and Intercultural Communication, 6*(2), 135-144. doi:10.1080/17513057.2013.776094

Lester, J. (2008). Performing gender in the workplace: Gender socialization, power and identity among women faculty members. *Community College Review, 35*(4), 277-305.

Schilt, K., & Connell, C. (2007). Do workplace gender transitions make gender trouble? *Gender, Work & Organization, 14*(6), 596-618.

Schilt, K., & Wiswall, M. (2008). Before and after: Gender transitions, human capital and workplace experiences. *Journal of Economic Analysis & Policy, 8*(1), Article 39.

Taranowski, C. J. (2008). Transsexual employees in the workplace. *Journal of Workplace Behavioural Health, 23*(4), 467-477. doi:10.1080/15555240802540186

Turkewitz, J. (2012, Jun 21). Transgender rights in the workplace are still unclear. *The Atlantic.* Retrieved from http://www.theatlantic.com/national/archive/2012/06/transgender-rights-in-the-workplace-are-still-unclear/258822/.

Walworth, J. (2003). Managing transexual transition in the workplace. Retrieved from http://www.gendersanity.com_

West, C., & Zimmerman, D. (1987). Doing gender. *Gender and Society, 1*(2), 125-151.

Land of Milk and Honey? Lesbian Families' Experiences of Breastfeeding

Phyllis L. F. Rippeyoung and Laurel Falconi

The last time I (Rippeyoung) was at this conference, with co-author Mary C. Noonan, I was looking at how breastfeeding influences father involvement in infant care (Rippeyoung & Noonan, 2012). What we found was that when children are breastfed, dads tend to do less infant care (although many of the effects disappear by the time the children are 2). A question that was nagging at me, though, was whether these effects are a result of breastfeeding, per se, or if they are result of patriarchal family structures. I wondered if we would find the same pattern if there were no men in the house, which led me to examine the infant feeding experiences of lesbian households.

Although lesbian/queer families represent a small fraction of all families, their minority status has the potential to illuminate many significant theoretical questions. Drawing on Black feminist sociologist Patricia Hill Collins' (1986) concept of the "outsider-within," Gabb (2004) argues that;

> From off-centre, marginal locations, "other" sexualities destabilise the taken-for-granted centrality of heterosexuality, and the binary logic that underpins this institution [...] This does not bestow innate objectivity on "others," but situates other-ness as a strate-

gic position from which to challenge the naturalising discourses and normative assumptions that construct traditional categories of being (p. 403).

In other words, we can better understand if the "typical" is inherently "natural" by exploring the experiences of those who fall outside the norm. Breastfeeding is replete with assumptions of its "naturalness." Since lesbian families have the potential to create multiple and creative ways of organizing their families, we can better see whether infant feeding practices make an inevitably rigid impact on how life with a baby is organized, or if the practices we see, *writ large,* are simply a function of preference, habit, culture, or tradition.

To answer some of these questions, I carried out a pilot study from November, 2011 to April, 2012, using qualitative interviews and a short survey of six families in Canada and the United States. Seven birth mothers (two of whom were partnered with each other, and therefore are both birth mothers and partners), and three non-birth-mother mothers were included in my sample (we do not have partner data from two of the birth mothers). Three families were Canadian and three were American. Two respondents self-identified as Jewish, one as Mexican-American, and the rest self-identified as White or Caucasian. All were legally partnered or married, and all were openly and unapologetically lesbian. Eight women had at least a Bachelor's degree, one had an MA, and another a PhD at the time of the interview. Nine had professional careers (notably, two were midwives), and one was a stay-at-home-mom (although, after the interview, she began an MA in English). Pseudonyms were used for all women.

Although the interviews were organized around an interview guide, the end of every interview included an open-ended question asking if she had something to say that had not yet come up. In analysing the data, we used a grounded-theory approach, allowing the women's experiences to speak before any theories were imposed upon them. We organized the research around four main emergent themes; challenges getting started breastfeeding; lesbian identity and infant feeding; gender, fairness, and the division of labor; and the importance of supportive partners.

There was much diversity in the breastfeeding experiences of this relatively homogenous group of socioeconomically privileged women. All but one woman was able to breastfeed "successfully." Notably, the woman who was least successful had everything in place to be the most successful (she was a midwife who had helped her partner breastfeed successfully past a year and a half, and was connected to many breastfeeding support professionals). Some felt empowered by breastfeeding, and that breastfeeding made their lives better. Some felt controlled by it, but were glad they did it. One became so depressed by it that she spent her days wishing it was time to go to sleep.

All mothers first stated that their being a lesbian had little to do with their breastfeeding, and yet, they all noted ways in which their identities as lesbians intersected with their mothering identities. For the more "femme" mothers, they were often assumed to be straight. The one more "butch" mother experienced the surprise of others when she nursed her child, as her partner was assumed to be the birth mother. One mother found La Leche League meetings to be helpful for infant feeding, but frustrating when the other mothers assumed she "had it so easy" since she was not partnered with a man.

All of the women noted that while breastfeeding, the breastfeeding mother was more likely to be the "carer" or the nurturer, although some claimed that they believed it had to do with who was the birth mom, rather than the type of feeding. Although there is merit to their argument, the couple that had the most overlap of nurturing care was in the couple where a child was fully weaned to a bottle at 4 months.

Overall, the diversity amidst relative homogeneity points to the ways in which breastfeeding needs supporting. Most of the women, in the beginning, had struggles, but many were able to breastfeed for more than a year, and many of those found the experience transformative in the most positive ways. They all said that they were able to do this due to the help of their supportive partners, parents, friends, midwives, and lactation consultants who made this possible.

At the same time, there were two women who had very negative experiences. One could not produce milk despite heroic efforts and having everything in place to be able to do it. She cried in the interview, thinking about her inability to breastfeed, even though she repeatedly said that she was okay with having stopped. The other, despite having had a very positive experience nursing her first child, found that for whatever reason, her very difficult second child made the process nearly unbearable. She explained that until she quit nursing, she was "in a very dark place."

What emerged from most of these women's stories were interconnected webs of love, support, comfort, and care, interspersed with frustrations, resentments, pain, and new self-insights. In other words, these mothers were, in many ways, like most mothers I have met. Nonetheless, their unique status as lesbians helps us to see beyond taken for granted assumptions about heteronormative-family life. Although lesbian families may not always find themselves in a blissful and divine land of milk and honey, the particular families I interviewed shine a light on the edges of assumptions and make it clear that mother and infant care go far beyond just what goes into babies' bellies.

References

Collins, P. H. (1986). Learning from the outsider within: The sociological significance of black feminist thought. *Social Problems, 33*(6), S14-S32.

Gabb, J. (2004). "I could eat my baby to bits": Passion and desire in lesbian mother-children love. *Gender, Place & Culture: A Journal of Feminist Geography, 11*(3), 399-415.

Rippeyoung, P. L. F., & Noonan, M. C. (2012). Breastfeeding and the gendering of infant care. In P. H. Smith, B. L. Hausman, and M. Labbok (Eds.), *Beyond Health, Beyond Choice: Breastfeeding Constraints and Realities* (pp. 133-143). New Brunswick, NJ: Rutgers University Press.

Forging Partnerships within the Health Care Community

Central to the consideration of breastfeeding and feminism is the reality of the positive health outcomes associated with breastfeeding. This chapter focusses first on issues that arise in the practice of breastfeeding support, and then on issues related to support by providers.

Section IIIa

Issues in Breastfeeding Support: From Birth to Birthspacing

Lactation Interventions and Maternal Well-being: A Qualitative Study

Elizabeth Wierman

Overview

This presentation draws upon a qualitative analysis of 9 semi-structured interviews of women who delivered children in Washington State, and utilized lactation interventions within the first month postpartum, examining maternal efforts to breastfeed and exploring the relationship between postpartum lactation interventions and maternal wellbeing. The examination of the relationship between lactation interventions and maternal wellbeing is a major contribution of this study. Interdisciplinary in nature, this research has implications for social work, as well as public health, and medicine.

Background

Contemporary culture idealizes and politicizes breastfeeding, sending a strong message that breastfeeding is a value to aspire to (Wolf, 2007; Avishai, 2007). Multiple studies have found that women experience enormous pressure to breastfeed, influenced by a larger ideology of mothering that establishes what it means to be a good mother (McDonald, Amir, & Davey, 2011; Andrews & Knaak, 2013; Knaak, 2010; Avishai, 2007). Influenced by an institution of motherhood that is expert guided and endorsed (Andrews & Knaak, 2013; Knaak, 2010), maternal decisions to breastfeed are guided by the belief that good mothers put their baby's health before their own (McDonald et al., 2011), operating within a context that does not take into account maternal health and wellbeing.

Despite the extensive body of research on breastfeeding, there is little research on the association between the use of intensive lactation services (e.g., use of lactation consultants, hospital-grade breast pumps, nipple shields, herbal supplements, etc.), and maternal wellbeing. While some research has explored the impact of breast pumps on breastfeeding (Buckley, 2009), and the ramification of nipple pain on maternal mood, sleep, and general activity (McClellan et al., 2012), few studies examine the effect of the multitude of lactation interventions currently used, nor do they emphasize maternal wellbeing as an outcome in evaluating the efficacy of such interventions.

This presentation seeks to fill this gap by focusing on maternal efforts to breastfeed, and exploring the relationship between postpartum lactation interventions and maternal wellbeing. This research draws upon a qualitative analysis of nine semi-structured interviews of women who utilized lactation interventions within the first month postpartum. Due to the lack of research on the complex interplay between lactation interventions and maternal wellbeing, an exploratory approach was used in an effort to create a framework that can inform future research and policy.

Method

This study uses a phenomenological approach to qualitative data analysis, in conjunction with a secondary analysis through review in QSR NVivo 10 software. Participants were recruited through two recruitment strategies; dissemination of a flier through the University of Washington's School of Social Work ,and through snowball sampling (i.e., the principal investigator asked women, such as fellow students at the University of Washington, acquaintances, and coworkers to participate and refer other participants).

Inclusion criteria included women aged 18 to 48 who gave birth, while age 18 to 38, in the time period of 01/01/2003 through 05/01/2013, and thereafter utilized lactation interventions within her first month (≤31 days) postpartum, gave birth, and received lactation services in Washington State. Currently pregnant women were excluded.

Each participant was interviewed for 45 to 60 minutes, utilizing a set of standardized interview questions and follow-up questions as appropriate. Interviews were recorded and transcribed. Participants were randomly assigned pseudonyms. Informed consent was obtained from all participants in accordance with the University of Washington's Institutional Review Board.

Results

While most study participants reported experiencing similar obstacles to breastfeeding (difficulty with infant latch, nipple position and pain, milk supply, and time), all participants reported utilizing three or more lactation interventions. The average number of lactation interventions utilized was five, and the most frequently utilized interventions were lactation consultants, breast pumps, nipple shields, and herbal supplements. Participants reported learning about lactation interventions from multiple sources, including medical professionals (e.g., lactation consultants, midwives, and doctors), family (typically mothers and/or sisters), books, and online resources.

While not all participants reported a negative connection between the use of lactation interventions and their wellbeing, some participants noted significant physical and/or psychological symptoms. Several participants reported experiencing pain as a result of continued breastfeeding, despite challenges. Other reported depression, anxiety, stress, sadness, a general state of feeling overwhelmed, as well as episodes of crying.

When asked why they continued to breastfeed, utilizing lactation interventions despite emotional and physical pain, study participants reported feeling pressure to breastfeed, some noting a culture of "breast is best," where mothers who struggle to breastfeed feel that they are failures at motherhood. The following quotes are extracted from interviews with two participants.

> Lauren: "So there is kind of this competitiveness undertone to, 'are you mom enough?' How mom are you? I feel like breastfeeding has become a part of that kind of image, and persona, and mark of how much of a mom are you?"

> Geneva: "[...] definitely breastfeeding fits in with that model of the 'good mom,' and I think that is a myth that needs to be dispelled."

Others participants experienced guilt, embarrassment, and shame around their inability to exclusively breastfeed, reporting perceived pressure to breastfeed at any cost. The following quotes are extracted from interviews with two participants.

> Esther: "But I think you hear the message like, this [breastfeeding] is kinda it, and if you don't do this, you are a failure."

> Freda: "A lot of my friends just couldn't believe that I would stop nursing my second child after only a few weeks of trying, and it was hard. I felt really judged."

Discussion

A culture of breastfeeding that is part and parcel of a larger ideology of motherhood has become firmly established. As a result, more and more women utilize lactation interventions to promote breastfeeding. However, maternal efforts to breastfeed in the face of obstacles are often due to societal pressures, and may be to the detriment of maternal wellbeing. Additionally, the current culture of breastfeeding has pitted women against one another, exemplifying a type of internalized oppression. More research is needed to thoroughly examine the impetus for use of lactation interventions, and to help identify strategies for eliminating the negative stigma associated with not breastfeeding. Future studies may benefit from a mixed-methods approach in order to more fully quantify the connection between lactation interventions on maternal wellbeing, as well as identify strategies to promote more empowering breastfeeding support for lactating mothers.

References

Andrews, T., & Knaak, S. (2013). Medicalized mothering: Experiences with breastfeeding in Canada and Corway. *The Sociological Review, 61*(1), 88-110.

Avishai, O. (2007). Managing the lactating body: The breast-feeding project and privileged motherhood. *Qualitative Sociology, 30*(2), 135-152.

Buckley, K. M. (2009). A double-edged sword: Lactation consultants' perceptions of the impact of breast pumps on the practice of breastfeeding. *Journal of Perinatal Education, 18*(2), 13-22. doi:10.1624/105812409X426297; 10.1624/105812409X426297

Knaak, S. J. (2010). Contextualising risk, constructing choice: Breastfeeding and good mothering in risk society. *Health, Risk, & Society, 12*(4), 345-355.

McClellan, H. L., Hepworth, A. R., Garbin, C. P., Rowan, M. K., Deacon, J., Hartmann, P. E., et al. (2012). Nipple pain during breastfeeding with or without visible trauma. *Journal of Human Lactation28*(4), 511-521. doi:10.1177/0890334412444464; 10.1177/0890334412444464

McDonald, K., Amir, L. H., & Davey, M. A. (2011). Maternal bodies and medicines: A commentary on risk and decision-making of pregnant and breastfeeding women and health professionals. *BMC Public Health, 11*(Suppl 5), S5-2458-11-S5-S5. doi:10.1186/1471-2458-11-S5-S5; 10.1186/1471-2458-11-S5-S5

Wolf, J. B. (2007). Is breast really best? Risk and total motherhood in the national breastfeeding awareness campaign. *Journal of Health Politics, Policy and Law, 32*(4), 595-636. doi:10.1215/03616878-2007-018

CHAPTER 17

Breastfeeding Practices and Mode of Delivery

Hira Palla and Panagiota Kitsantas

Abstract

B *ackground/Purpose:* Mode of delivery can influence breastfeeding
outcomes. The purpose of this study was to compare early
breastfeeding practices, including initiation, exclusivity, and intensity
of breastfeeding among women who had an unplanned caesarean
section (C-section), a planned C-section, vaginal-induced delivery,
and a vaginal, but not induced delivery. Associations between several
prenatal factors, family/peer influence, and early breastfeeding practices were assessed for these groups of women.

Method: Data was obtained from the Infant Feeding Practices Study
II (*N* = 2551), a longitudinal, national survey administered by the U.S.
Food and Drug Administration and Centers for Disease Control and
Prevention that followed women from pregnancy to 1 year postpartum.
Descriptive statistics and chi-square analysis were conducted.

Results: During the prenatal period, when asked about their plan
to feed their baby, women with a planned cesarean were less likely to
report a plan of exclusively breastfeeding their child (52.1%). Women
with an unplanned cesarean were less likely to exclusively breastfeed
their baby at 2 months postpartum (30.5%). Among the women who
were breastfeeding at 2 months, those who underwent vaginally
induced labor had the lowest breastfeeding intensity (35.6%), followed

closely by women who had a cesarean (35.1%). Women with a planned cesarean were the least likely to report a clinician's support for breast-feeding. They were more likely to report that family members (40.8%) and clinicians (20.9%) supported formula, or the use of a combination of formula and human milk.

Conclusions: Breastfeeding practices among women with a cesarean fell short of clinical-practice guidelines for infant-feeding behaviors. Since hospital stay is known to be a critical period for the establishment of breastfeeding, interventions should focus on improving breastfeeding support in hospitals, particularly among women who have had a planned cesarean and vaginally induced labor.

Introduction

Despite the known benefits of nourishing infants exclusively with mother's milk, the rates of breastfeeding initiation, continuation, and exclusive breastfeeding during the first few months of infancy are lower than expected among U.S. mothers (Ahluwalia, Li, & Morrow, 2012). Mothers and infants' experiences during labor and delivery may affect lactation and breastfeeding outcomes. Vaginally induced birth has been associated with not initiating breastfeeding (Leung, Lam, & Ho, 2002). Furthermore, cesarean deliveries (cesareans) have been associated with lower initiation rates, shorter breastfeeding duration rate, and lower success in breastfeeding, compared to undergoing a vaginal delivery (Dewey, Nommsen-Rivers, Heinig, & Cohen, 2003 Zanardo et al., 2010). This may be due to delays in mother/infant skin-to-skin contact, mother's post-surgery physical complications, and effects of anesthetics (Kearney, Cronenwett, & Reinhardt, 1990; Dennis, 2002). In addition to mode of delivery, other factors that may influence breastfeeding initiation and duration include problems encountered during nursing, availability of support systems, mother's sociocultural and economic situation, and the recommendations and attitudes of family, peers, and health professionals (Cakmak & Kuguoglu, 2007; Kornides & Kitsantas, 2013).

Previous studies that have examined the relationship between mode of delivery and breastfeeding outcomes had either small sample sizes or were confined to a single geographic location (Prior et al., 2012). The purpose of the present study was to evaluate early breast-feeding practices, including initiation, exclusivity, and intensity of breastfeeding in the first 2 months of infant age among women who had an unplanned cesarean , a planned cesarean , vaginal induced delivery, and a vaginal, but not induced delivery using a large, nation-ally distributed U.S. population. Further, we assessed relationships between breastfeeding support by family, peers, clinicians, and breast-feeding patterns during the first 2 months.

Method

Data was obtained from the Infant Feeding Practices Study II (IFPS II), a longitudinal national survey administered by the U.S. Food and Drug Administration and Centers for Disease Control and Prevention that followed women from pregnancy to 1 year postpartum. In IFPS II, inclusion criteria required that the infant was born after 35 weeks gestation, weighed at least 5 lbs., was a singleton, and was not hospi-talized for longer than 3 days following birth (Fein, Labiner-Wolfe, Shealy, Chen, & Grummer-Strawn, 2008). Approximately 4,900 women participated at the beginning of the study. The sample size for this study, however, was reduced for early infant feeding behaviors (2-months infant age) due to follow up loss and missing data on the main variables (N= 2,551). For certain variables, including reasons for not initiating breastfeeding, the sample size was reduced to 414 women.

Mode of delivery, which includes the categories of vaginal, not-in-duced labor, vaginally induced labor, planned caesarean section, and unplanned caesarean section, was the main exposure variable.

Outcome variables included breastfeeding patterns during first 2 months (if the baby was ever breastfed, exclusive breastfeeding at infant age 2 months, and breastfeeding intensity). Breastfeeding intensity was constructed by averaging the proportion of human milk to the total milk diet (including human milk, formula, cow's milk, other milk) that the baby received on a daily basis; a categorical variable was created with two levels: low defined as < 20% of milk feedings being human milk, and medium/high defined as ≥20% of milk feedings being human milk. Clinician and family opinions about breastfeeding, number of friends who breastfed, plan to breastfeed, breastfeeding support during neonatal period from professionals, lactation consultant, nurse, and family members were assessed. Sources of breastfeeding information, such as information received from nurse lactation consultant, relatives/friends, and birthing/baby care classes during the first 2 months were also included in the analyses. Further important reasons for not initiating breastfeeding in neonatal period were assessed. Other variables included mother's age, education, marital status, prenatal smoking, and pre-pregnancy BMI. Descriptive statistics and chi-square analysis were conducted.

Results

Table 1 presents the distribution of prenatal sample sociodemographic characteristics by mode of delivery. We observed that women who were at least 34 years old were more likely to have a planned cesarean (23.7%), and less likely to have a vaginally induced delivery (11.5%). Furthermore, women who had a planned cesareans were significantly more likely to be BMI >30 (41.4%) and married (85.6%).

Table 2 presents breastfeeding patterns during the first 2 months, stratified by the mode of delivery. Twenty-percent of women who had planned cesareans did not initiate breastfeeding, and this was the lowest breastfeeding initiation rate in the sample. Furthermore, women who had an unplanned cesarean were less likely to exclusively breastfeed their baby at 2 months (30.5%). Among women who had breastfed their baby at 2 months, a higher proportion of those who underwent vaginally induced labor had the lowest breastfeeding intensity (35.6%), followed closely by women who had unplanned cesareans (35.1%).

Table 3 provides information on the associations between breastfeeding attitude and support variables with mode of delivery. A significantly higher proportion of women who did not undergo vaginally induced labor had families who supported breastfeeding only (52.4%). On the other hand, women who had a planned cesarean had a higher likelihood of having family members (40.8%) and clinicians (20.9%) who supported formula, or the use of a combination of formula and human milk. Women who had a planned cesarean were significantly less likely to report a plan to exclusively breastfeed their child (52.1%), and more likely to indicate their plan to feed their infant formula only (18.8%). A higher proportion of women who underwent vaginally induced labor planned to use a combination of formula and human milk (24.9%).

Table 4 provides information on breastfeeding support in neonatal period and month 2 period stratified by mode of delivery. A significantly higher proportion of women with planned cesareans received the least professional breastfeeding support. This group was also less likely to receive breastfeeding information from relatives/friends (48.9%). Women who underwent vaginally induced labor were less likely to be provided with breastfeeding information from both a midwife/nurse practitioner (59.3%), and a birthing or baby-care class (29.4%).

Table 5 provides information on the reasons for not initiating breastfeeding in the neonatal period stratified by mode of delivery. Women who had an unplanned cesarean were more likely to cite medical issues (45.8%), and having work or school (59.6%), while women who underwent a vaginal delivery cited inconvenience (58.6%), wanting to leave the baby for hours at a time (45.7%), finding formula to be the same or better compared to human milk (71%), wanting someone else to feed the baby (55%), and discouragement from family members (16.9%) as important reasons. A higher proportion of women who underwent vaginally induced labor reported their intention to make at least three lifestyle changes (16%) as important reasons for not initiating breastfeeding.

Discussion

Factors associated with having a cesarean can serve as obstacles in initiating breastfeeding (Rowe-Murray & Fisher, 2002). Early contact between mothers and infants in the first few hours postpartum is important for forming a mother-infant interaction, as well as crucial for breastfeeding success. However, operative-care routines with post-caesarean delivery can delay mothers from holding their infants, and disrupt bonding between mother and infant, all this negatively affecting breastfeeding initiation (Prior et al., 2012). Along with mode of delivery, other factors, such as family and clinician opinions, as well as work, may influence the mother's infant-feeding choice.

Our findings indicate that women who had a planned cesarean were less likely to receive breastfeeding support from family members and clinicians during prenatal period, as well as inadequate breast-feeding information from relatives/friends during month 2. This may explain why a significantly lower proportion of this group initiated breastfeeding and suggests that family and health providers' opinion can have a significant influence on the mother's decision to breast-feed (Kornides & Kitsantas, 2013). We also found that those who are more likely to initiate breastfeeding, as well as exclusively breastfeed at 2 months postpartum, also tended to have more friends who had breastfed. This suggests that peers may also influence a mother's decision to breastfeed.

Furthermore, women who had an unplanned cesarean were more likely to find work or school as major obstacles in initiating breastfeeding during neonatal period. Additionally, this group was also less likely to exclusively breastfeed at 2 months compared to women who underwent other modes of delivery. Having more breastfeeding support at the workplace by dedicating facilities where mothers can express and store milk has been found to be helpful in increasing breastfeeding initiation and exclusive breastfeeding rates (Smith et al., 2013).

In conclusion, this study provides evidence that infant-feeding practices differ among women have to undergo different modes of delivery. Breastfeeding practices among women with a cesarean fell short of clinical practice guidelines for infant-feeding behaviors. Our results suggest that women who had a cesarean may need extra encouragement from family members and clinicians in initiating breastfeeding, as well as adequate breastfeeding support through month 2 postpartum. Since hospital stay is known to be a critical period for the establishment of breastfeeding, breastfeeding interventions should focus on improving breastfeeding support in hospitals, particularly among women who have had a planned cesarean. Due to our sample being limited to women with high educational levels and socioeconomic status, future replication studies should include population-based representation of Black and Hispanic mother-infant dyads of low-income mothers.

References

Ahluwalia, I., Li, R., & Morrow, B. (2012). Breastfeeding practices: Does method of delivery really matter? *Maternal and Child Health Journal, 16*(2),. 231-237.

Cakmak, H., & Kuguoglu, S. (2007). Comparison of the breastfeeding patterns of mothers who delivered their babies per vagina and via cesarean section: An observational study using the LATCH breastfeeding charting system. *International Journal of Nursing Studies, 44*(7).

Dennis, C. L. (2002). Breastfeeding initiation and duration: A 1990-2000 literature review. *Journal of Obstetric, Gynecologic, & Neonatal Nursing, 31*(1), 12-32.

Dewey, K., Nommsen-Rivers, L., Heinig, J., & Cohen, R. (2003). Risk factors for suboptimal infant breastfeeding behavior, delayed onset of lactation, and excess neonatal weight loss. *Pediatrics, 112*(3), 607-619.

Fein, S. B., Labiner-Wolfe, J., Shealy, K. R., Chen, J., & Grummer-Strawn, L. M. (2008). Infant feeding practices study II: Study methods. *Pediatrics, 122*, S28-S35.

Kearney, M., Cronenwett, L., & Reinhardt, R. (1990). Caesarean delivery and breastfeeding outcomes. *Birth, 17*(2), 97-103.

Kornides, M., & Kitsantas, P. (2013). Evaluation of breastfeeding promotion, support, and knowledge of benefits on breastfeeding outcomes. *Journal of Child Health Care, 17*(3), 264-273.

Leung, G. M., Lam, T. H., & Ho, L. M. (2002). Breast-feeding and its relation to smoking and mode of delivery. *Obstetrics & Gynecology, 99*(5), 785-794.

Prior, E., Santhakumaran, S., Gale, C., Philipps, L. H., Modi, N., & Hyde, M. J. (2012). Breastfeeding after cesarean delivery: A systematic review and meta-analysis of world literature. *The American Journal of Clinical Nutrition, 95*(5), 1113-1135.

Rowe-Murray, H. J., & Fisher, J. R. (2002). Baby-friendly hospital practices: Cesarean section is a persistent barrier to early initiation of breastfeeding. *Birth, 29*(2), 124-131.

Smith, J. P., McIntyre, E., Craig, L., Javanparast, S., Strazdins, L., & Mortensen, K. (2013). Workplace support, breastfeeding and health. *Family Matters, 93*(58), Retrieved from https://aifs.gov.au/publications/family-matters/issue-93/workplace-support-breastfeeding-and-health.

Zanardo, V., Svegliado, G., Cavallin, F., Giustardi, A., Cosmi, E., Litta, P., & Trevisanuto, D. (2010). Elective cesarean delivery: Does it have a negative effect on breastfeeding? *Birth, 37*(4), 275-279.

Table 1

Distribution of Prenatal Sample Sociodemographic Characteristics by Mode of Delivery

Characteristics	Vaginally, not induced %	Vaginally & induced %	Planned C-section %	Unplanned C-section %	P-value
Mother's age					0.00
18-24 years	60.4	64.8	64.0	51.0	
25-34 years	25.5	23.7	12.3	28.4	
≥34 years	14.0	11.5	23.7	20.7	
Mother's education					0.20
High school or less	20.5	23.4	18.8	18.7	
Some college	39.3	40.8	41.7	39.9	
4-year college or more	40.2	38.5	39.5	41.4	
Maternal smoking					0.85
Non-smoker	90.2	90.5	90.1	89.0	
Smoker	9.8	9.5	9.9	11.0	
Marital status					0.00
Married	77.6	79.8	85.6	72.4	
Widowed/Divorced/ Separated	4.5	4.7	4.1	3.7	
Never Married	17.9	15.5	10.3	23.8	
Pre-pregnancy BMI					0.00
Normal Weight	51.7	47.3	36.2	38.4	
Underweight	13.9	10.8	7.5	5.3	
BMI 26-29	14.4	14.8	15.0	17.9	
BMI >30	20.1	27.2	41.4	38.4	

Table 2

Breastfeeding Patterns during the First Two Months by Mode of Delivery

	Vaginally not induced %	Vaginally & induced %	Planned C-section %	Unplanned C-section %	P-value
Baby was ever breastfed					0.00
Breastfed	87.0	85.4	80.0	86.0	
Not Breastfed	13.0	14.6	20.0	14.0	
Exclusive breast-feeding at 2-months infant age					0.00
No	55.3	65.7	63.7	69.5	
Yes	44.7	34.3	36.3	30.5	
Breastfeeding intensity at 2-months infant age					0.00
Low	24.7	35.6	34.3	35.1	
Medium/High	75.3	64.4	65.7	64.9	

Table 3

Breastfeeding Attitudes and Support by Mode of Delivery

Characteristics	Vaginally not induced %	Vaginally & induced %	Planned C-section %	Unplanned C-section %	p-value
Clinician opinion					0.02
Formula only or combination of formula and breastfeeding	14.6	15.8	20.9	15.0	
Breastfeeding only	48.1	45.5	40.2	46.4	
No opinion	37.3	38.7	38.8	38.6	
Family opinion					0.01
BF only	52.4	51.2	42.5	49.3	
No opinion	15.1	15.2	16.7	16.4	
Formula only or both	32.4	33.6	40.8	34.3	
Friends who breastfed					0.01
1-2	20.9	22.8	21.8	23.3	
3-5	26.2	26.8	29.8	31.7	
At least 5	39.5	35.7	35.7	27.5	
Plan to feed the baby					0.00
Breastfeeding only	62.7	60.1	52.1	60.5	
formula only	12.2	12.2	18.8	12.7	
BF and formula	21.8	24.9	24.5	22.7	
Don't know yet	3.3	2.9	4.5	4.1	

Table 4

Breastfeeding Support in Neonatal and Month 2 Periods by Mode of Delivery

Sources of Breastfeeding Support	Vaginally not induced %	Vaginally & induced %	Planned C-section %	Unplanned C-section %	p-value
Professional Breast-feeding Support					0.00
None to one	95.4	96.9	99.3	98.5	
At least 2	4.6	3.1	.7	1.5	
Lactation consultant helped with breast-feeding	58	58.9	65.8	70.3	0.00
Family member helped with breastfeeding	12.4	15	12.5	19.4	0.03
Nurse/nurse midwife/ Nurse practitioner provided information about breastfeeding	64.4	59.3	61.3	69.3	0.02
Lactation consultant provided information about breastfeeding	56.5	61.4	63	70.3	0.00
Relatives/friends provided information about breastfeeding	56	51	48.9	62.5	0.00
Birthing or baby care class provided information about breastfeeding	35	29.4	32	40.3	0.01

Table 5

Reasons for Not Initiating Breastfeeding in the Neonatal Period by Mode of Delivery

Important Reasons	Vaginally not induced %	Vaginally & induced %	Planned C-section %	Unplanned C-section %	P-value
Medical reasons*	26.4	32.6	29.9	45.8	0.09
Formula is same or better	71.0	57.2	69.3	61.2	0.07
Inconvenience	58.6	51.8	48.2	49.0	0.40
Wanted to leave baby hours at a time	45.7	41.9	31.4	29.4	0.06
Lifestyle changes**					0.15
1-2 lifestyle changes	37	32.1	25.9	20.4	
3 or more lifestyle changes	15.2	16	10.	12.2	
Have work or school	46.5	40.3	34.1	59.6	0.02
Someone else feed the baby***	55	51.1	40.7	54.2	0.19
Family reasons****	16.9	11.9	10.3	4	0.09

* Medical Reasons includes mother was sick or on medication.

**Lifestyle changes include wanted to go on a weight loss diet, go back to original diet, wanted to smoke, mother wanted body back to herself, wanted to use incompatible contraception.

***Someone else feed the baby includes mother wanted someone else to feed baby and someone else wanted to feed baby.

**** Family reasons include baby's grandmother didn't want her to breastfeed and baby's father didn't want her to breastfeed.

Breastfeeding for Preterm Babies in NICU

Yeon Bai

Abstract

Premature babies in NICU face a higher risk of infection because their immune systems are particularly immature. Live cells in human milk that protect babies from infection can be even more important for them. Mothers of preterm babies in NICU encounter emotional and physical challenges associated with the birth of vulnerable premature babies, leaving them in need of strong support for breastfeeding during and after NICU stay. A hospital in central New Jersey launched a project with the purpose of improving breastfeeding rates and behaviors among mothers of premature babies in NICU with the March of Dimes grant.

Since August, 2012, a lactation consultant solely dedicated to NICU population was hired for the hospital. The lactation consultant visits every NICU baby within 24 hours of admission to support breastfeeding, log breastfeeding status and any breastfeeding concerns of mothers, and enable mothers to express milk manually and use a pump, position properly for nursing, and troubleshoot. She follows up with mothers at discharge, 14 days of life, and 1 week after discharge from the hospital.

After the project completion in December, 2013, breastfeeding initiation rates increased to 98.9% compared to 82% before the project implementation (z=7.34, p<0.001). The breastfeeding rate at discharge was 61.4%, and 14 days of life was 58.9%. The breastfeeding rate at 1 week after discharge is 51.8%. Mothers mentioned that "good milk supply" (35.8%) and "good latch" (27.4%) were facilitators for breastfeeding. "Low milk supply" (46%) was frequently mentioned for the barrier. Interestingly, "pumping" was mentioned as both facilitator (4.6%) and barrier (5.1%).

The rates could stabilize as the project progresses, but further examination is needed to address the barriers mentioned, and to identify other factors associated with decreased breastfeeding continuation rates from a higher breastfeeding initiation rate in this hospital.

Background

Currently, one in eight babies is born prematurely every year in the U.S. (U.S. Department of Health and Human Services [HHS], 2011). Premature babies are at a higher risk for medical problems because their immune systems are particularly immature. Human milk not only provides perfect nutrition for all babies, but also contains antibodies and other substances that protect babies from disease. These benefits of human milk are even more important for premature babies. Preterm babies who are breastfed are found to have stayed in the hospital for a shorter duration and have been positively affected regarding their long-term mental and motor development, as well as visual acuity (Vohr et al., 2007).

Although the overall breastfeeding initiation rates in the U.S. have improved steadily, the rates are lower among mothers of premature babies. Currently, 59% to 70% of mothers initiate breastfeeding for their preterm babies born between 34 and 37 weeks gestation, yet the continuation of breastfeeding beyond 4 weeks is less than that for term babies (Radke, 2011). Premature babies are more likely to be in NICU (Neonatal Intensive Care Unit), and separated from mothers for medical issues. Studies report that the reasons for suboptimal breast-feeding rates among NICU mothers include inconsistent, inaccurate information, and lack of support by health care professionals (Jaeger, Lawson, & Filteau, 1997).

Mothers of preterm babies in NICU encounter emotional and physical challenge associated with the birth of vulnerable premature babies, leaving them in need of strong support for breastfeeding during and after NICU stay (Campbell & Gutman, 2007). Successful breastfeeding initiation depends on experiences in the hospital, as well as access to instruction on lactation from breastfeeding experts, particularly in the early postpartum period. A hospital in central New Jersey launched a breastfeeding promotion program with the purpose of improving breastfeeding rates and behaviors among mothers of premature babies in NICU. This study was conducted to evaluate the impact of this program.

Method

The duration of the promotion program was September, 2012 to December, 2013. Specific aims of the project were: 1) increase breastfeeding initiation in NICU, 2) increase breastfeeding continuation at hospital discharge and at 14 days of life, and 3) examine barriers and facilitators of breastfeeding among mothers in NICU.

A lactation consultant solely dedicated to NICU population was hired for the hospital to implement the program. The consultant worked 32 hours per week, distributing her work hours for 5 days a week. She visited all infants in NICU within 24 hours of their admission, and offered breastfeeding support and education. After the initial visit, she made daily rounds on the mothers to follow up with breastfeeding and further assistance. During their hospital stay, mothers were also inquired about barriers and facilitators of breastfeeding. In addition, the consultant followed up with mothers after discharge to assist mothers with home breastfeeding, and to measure breastfeeding continuation.

The goal of breastfeeding education was to help mothers become independent with breastfeeding. The consultant discussed kangaroo care with mothers at each individual consultation visit. Mothers were provided with kangaroo information in NICU welcome packet. Every NICU room was equipped with a reclining rocking chair and a mirror, as well as a double- electric breast pump, so that mothers can pump after kangaroo care. If pumping is needed, it is initiated within 6 hours of delivery, but the consultant taught manual expression so that mothers may get colostrum within the first hour after delivery. Mothers also received education on benefits of human milk, pumping technique and storage, hand hygiene, and sterilization pump parts. Using a bedside kardex, the consultant followed the breastfeeding progress with mothers (e.g., education topics covered, pumping technique progress, or their baby's readiness for direct nursing).

Evaluation was conducted at midpoints of the program and at the end of the implementation. The proportions of mothers who initiated breastfeeding during hospital stay, who continued breastfeeding at hospital discharge, at 14 days of life, and at 1-week post discharge were assessed and compared to the proportions before the program implementation using z-tests. Barriers and facilitators of breastfeeding were summarized to determine primary and common responses. The impact of the program was evaluated by comparing before and after the program implementation.

Results

A total of 304 postpartum mothers were served for the duration of this program. The mean birth weight of the infants was 2.62 ± 0.90 kg, and gestation age was 35.5 ± 3.82 weeks. The main impact of the program was the significant improvement in the exclusive breastfeeding initiation rate for NICU mothers compared to the baseline: 98.9% vs. 82% ($z=7.34$, $p<0.001$). The post-program exclusive breastfeeding rates at 14 days of life and at discharge were 58.9% and 61.4%, respectively. Continuation rates were significantly lower than the baseline ($p<0.001$). The breastfeeding rate measured at 1-week post-discharge was 51.8%, which was not compared to the baseline because no baseline rate was available.

Mothers of infants in NICU named "excellent and good milk supply" (35.8%) to be the number one facilitator of breastfeeding, followed by "good latch" (27.4%), and "breastfeeding support in NICU" (15.3%)." Also, mothers mentioned that "low milk supply" (46%) is the primary barrier of breastfeeding followed by "inconvenience" (10.7%). However, "pumping" was mentioned both as a facilitator (4.6%) and a barrier (5.1%).

Discussion

The success of this promotion program is in its impact on the rate of exclusive breastfeeding initiation, which is most likely due to the regular presence of the lactation consultation in NICU. Previous studies reported that breastfeeding support during hospital stay for preterm babies increased breastfeeding (Sisk, Lovelady, Dillard, & Gruber, 2006). Close monitoring of breastfeeding by the lactation consultant in this hospital had a positive influence on the breast-feeding initiation. Mothers in NICU are more vulnerable to terminate breastfeeding because of medical and emotional issues that come with the infant in NICU. Appropriate and timely support of breastfeeding is essential to help these mothers. By having the consultant regularly, mothers in this hospital were able to initiate breastfeeding.

The lactation consultant plays an important role in improving breastfeeding rates among mothers of infants in NICU. Many health care providers are not confident to provide effective and appropriate lactation care and services because they were not properly trained during their schooling. Effective lactation support is time intensive, with an average consultation lasting one hour, which can be a challenge for other providers. One study reported that the presence of a lactation consultant in NICU improved the breastfeeding rate to 50% from 36% (Castrucci, Hoover, Lim, & Maus, 2007). In hospitals, there was a 2.28 times increase in breastfeeding at discharge with the help of lactation consultants (Castrucci, Hoover, Lim, & Maus, 2006). It has been estimated that 72% of lactation care and services cannot be deferred to nursing or non-clinical staff. Our study supports this important role of the lactation consultant in breastfeeding success.

A recent study reported that "mothers of preterm babies who are admitted to the NICU are more likely to initiate and continue breastfeeding than mothers of infants placed in the well-baby nursery" (Colaizy & Morriss, 2008). Education and follow-ups are keys in the continuation of breastfeeding preterm infants after hospital discharge. There is an urgent need for a system for follow-ups because the current study also indicated that the breastfeeding rate at 1-week post-discharge has dropped to 51.8%, which can be prevented if there is an easy access to lactation care after discharge. In addition, breastfeeding prevalence for post-discharge can be further improved with the proper utilization of community-based peer counseling programs, which was established in the 1980s to support breastfeeding in the early weeks of postpartum.

Perception of milk supply was frequently cited concern for breastfeeding. Good milk supply was mentioned for a breastfeeding facilitator in this study. Low milk supply was mentioned most frequently for a barrier in this study as several other studies (Heinig et al., 2006). One national study found that about 50% of mothers cited low milk supply as their reason for stopping breastfeeding (Li, Fein, Chen, & Grummer-Strawn, 2008). Contributors to insufficient milk supply include infrequent feeding, poor breastfeeding techniques (Amir, 2006), lack of skin-to-skin contact, mismanaged supplementation, physiological distress, and infrequent breast stimulation (Campbell & Gutman, 2007). A lack of confidence in breastfeeding, or not understanding the normal physiology of lactation can also lead to the perception of an insufficient milk supply when, in fact, the quantity is enough to nurture the baby (Powers, 1999).

Moreover, breastfeeding preterm infants come with many issues. These preterm infants are often sleepier and have less muscle strength, causing them to have difficulty with latch, suck, and swallow (Lapillonne, O'Connor, Wang, & Rigo, 2013). Because of their prematurity, they are more likely to be separated from their mothers, and this separation further interferes with breastfeeding.

Another important finding of this study is the fact that mothers listed pumping as both facilitator and barrier. For some mothers of infants in NICU, pumping is a necessary process to maintain and supply human milk to the infant who cannot nurse directly. Since pumping may become an intensive workload for new mothers, it can add to the stress they already feel (Campbell & Gutman, 2007). Lactation consultant can help mothers view pumping positively: "providing human milk is a way of being connected despite separation," and "breastfeeding constitutes motherhood," as mothers reported in one study (Aagaard & Hall, 2008). Continued support in and out of hospital by lactation consultants and peer mothers is imperative in order to encourage and support mothers of preterm babies to initiate and sustain breastfeeding.

Acknowledgement

This study has been supported in part by March of Dimes, Lactation Consultants, and hospital staff.

References

Aagaard, H., & Hall, E. O. (2008). Mothers' experiences of having a preterm infant in the neonatal care unit: A meta-synthesis. *Journal of Pediatric Nursing, 23*(3), e26-e36.

Amir, L. H. (2006). Breastfeeding–managing "supply" difficulties. *Australian Family Physician, 35*(9), 686-689.

Campbell, S. H., & Gutman, C. (2007). A case study: Challenges of breastfeeding preterm infants. *AWHONN Lifelines, 10*(6), 490-497.

Castrucci, B. C., Hoover, K. L., Lim, S., & Maus, K. C. (2006). A comparison of breastfeeding rates in an urban birth cohort among women delivering infants at hospitals that employ and do not employ lactation consultants. *Journal of Public Health Management and Practice, 12*(6), 578-585.

Castrucci, B. C., Hoover, K. L., Lim, S., & Maus, K. C. (2007). Availability of lactation counseling services influences breastfeeding among infants admitted to neonatal intensive care units. *American Journal of Health Promotion, 21*(5), 410-415.

Colaizy, T. T., & Morriss, F.H. (2008). Positive effect of NICU admission on breastfeeding of preterm US infants in 2000 to 2003. *Journal of Perinatology, 28*, 505-510.

Heinig, M. J., Follett, J. R., Ishii, K. D., Kavanagh-Prochaska, K., Cohen, R., Panchula, J. (2006). Barriers to compliance with infant-feeding recommendations among low-income women. *Journal of Human Lactation, 22*(1), 27-38.

Jaeger, M., Lawson, M., & Filteau, S. (1997). The impact of prematurity and neonatal illness on the decision to breastfeed. *Journal of Advanced Nursing, 25*, 729-737.

Lapillonne, A., O'Connor, D. L., Wang, D., & Rigo, J. (2013). Nutritional recommendations for the late-preterm infant and the preterm infant after hospital discharge. *Journal of Pediatrics, 162*(Suppl. 3), S90-S100.

Li, R., Fein, S. B., Chen, J., & Grummer-Strawn, L. M. (2008). Why mothers stop breastfeeding: Mothers' self-reported reasons for stopping during the first year. *Pediatrics, 122*(Suppl. 2), S69-S76.

Powers, N. G. (1999). Slow weight gain and low milk supply in the breastfeeding dyad. *Clinics of Perinatology, 26*(2), 399-430.

Radke, J. V. (2011). The paradox of breastfeeding-associated morbidity among late preterm infants. *Journal of Obstetric, Gynecologic, and Neonatal Nursing, 40*, 9-24.

Sisk, P. M., Lovelady, C. A., Dillard, R. G., & Gruber, K. J. (2006). Lactation counseling for mothers of very low birth weight infants: Effect on maternal anxiety and infant intake of human milk. *Pediatrics, 117*(1), e67-e75.

U.S. Department of Health and Human Services. (2011). Healthy people 2020. *Objective MICH, 9*(1). Retrieved from http://www.healthypeople. gov/2020/topicsobjectives2020/objectiveslist.aspx?topicId=26

Vohr, B. R., Poindexter, B. B., Dusick, A. M., McKinley, L. T., Higgins, R. D., Langer, J. C., & Poole, W. K. (2007). Persistent beneficial effects of breast milk ingested in the neonatal intensive care unit on outcomes of extremely low birth weight infants at 30 months of age. *Pediatrics, 120*(4), e953-e959.

Opioid Use and Breastfeeding: Current Status and Promising Futures

Kathryn Webb and Laurie Meschke

Current Trends and Characteristics

The first portion of presentation will explore the trends and characteristics of breastfeeding for women in treatment for opioid use (National Institute on Drug Abuse, 2005). Addiction to opioids, including heroin and the misuse of prescription medications, such as morphine and oxycodone, is oftentimes treated with the use of methadone or buprenorphine to reduce withdrawal effects and reduce the likelihood of relapse. Of women, ages 15 to 44, 5.2% have used illicit drugs in the past month (Bauer et al., 2002), and 4.4% of pregnant women have reported illicit drug use in the past 30 days (Substance Abuse and Mental Health Services Administration, 2011).

Neonatal abstinence syndrome (NAS) is a diagnosable condition associated with prenatal exposure to illegal or prescription drugs (Jansson & Velez, 2012). Symptoms can vary by type of drug used, duration, and severity of drug use, maternal metabolism, infant metabolism, and duration of gestation. Symptoms of NAS include neurological excitability, GI dysfunction, and autonomic signs (American Academy of Pediatrics, 1998). The infant withdrawal can last from 48 hours to 4 weeks (Kandall et al., 1977). Annually, about 50,000 infants receive inpatient pharmacotherapy as NAS treatment associated with withdrawal (Backes et al., 2012). In relation to pharmacotherapy, human milk of mothers who are in treatment for opioid addiction has been related to reduced NAS symptoms for infants, although methadone in human milk is low (McCarthy & Posey, 2000) regardless of treatment dosage (Jansson et al., 2008).

Factors Affecting Breastfeeding

The second portion of the presentation will focus on factors associated with breastfeeding among women in treatment for opioid use. The decision to breastfeed, among this population, is complicated by personal challenges, social barriers, and cultural stigma. This presentation will highlight specific factors in all three areas beginning with personal challenges.

Among opiate users, low confidence and low levels of education are common. These personal factors interfere with seeking prenatal care and assistance for substance abuse (Alto & O'Connor, 2011). Both low self-esteem and low education are negatively correlated with breast-feeding success. Similarly, social disadvantage and economic hardship negatively impact breastfeeding. Women in treatment for opioid use often incur the cost of missed work days in order to attend therapy sessions (Alto & O'Connor, 2011). With low financial resources, they may temporarily live with family or friends who further expose them to the harmful drug culture. Formula-fed infants are more likely than breastfed infants to have younger, unemployed mothers, and live in socially disadvantaged situations (Abdel-Latif et al., 2006).

Personal challenges affecting mothers' ability to breastfeed also include medical contraindications to breastfeeding. Drug abusing women, and women in treatment for opioid use, are at an increased risk for HIV and Hepatitis C. While Hepatitis C is not contraindicated with breastfeeding, health professionals strongly discourage women with HIV living in developed countries from breastfeeding (ABM Clinical Protocol #21, 2009). Like HIV, polysubstance use is also a contraindication to breastfeeding. Cigarette smoking and relapse to illicit substance abuse are common among women in treatment for opioid use (Abdel-Latif et al., 2006; Abrahams et al., 2007). Also common are psychiatric disorders, which often require medications not conducive to breastfeeding (Abdel-Latif et al., 2006; ABM Clinical Protocol #21, 2009).

Quality and quantity of prenatal care is another personal factor affecting breastfeeding outcomes. Lack of prenatal care and/or failure to adhere to prenatal recommendations lowers breastfeeding education and success among women in treatment for opioid use. Low prenatal care also increases the likelihood of NAS in infants born to mothers in treatment (American College of Obstetricians and Gynecologists, 2012). There is evidence to suggest that breastfeeding reduces NAS symptoms; the two factors also seem to work bi-directionally. Infants with mild NAS may be more successful at breastfeeding than infants with severe NAS, who exhibit breathing, sucking, and swallowing difficulties.

Social factors affecting breastfeeding among women in treatment for opioid use include partner and peer drug abuse, domestic violence, and separation from partner or spouse. Living among friends and family who use illicit drugs increases a woman's risk for relapsing into opioid abuse. Drug abusing women are also more likely to experience domestic violence and single parenthood (Abdel-Latif et al., 2006). Breastfeeding rates are significantly lower among women without partner support than among women who have the approval and encouragement of their partners (Giugliani, Caiaffa, Vogelhut, Witter, & Perman, 1994).

The cultural stigma, and associated guilt and shame of drug addiction during pregnancy, may result in attempts to hide the drug use and/or hide the pregnancy until delivery. Women in treatment for opioid use may fear that seeking prenatal care will result in the loss of custody of their child or the monitoring of their homes, partners, children, etc. (Alto & O'Connor, 2011). Because low prenatal care is associated with low breastfeeding rates, societal pressures that keep women from seeking care may prevent mothers in treatment for opioid use from breastfeeding successfully.

Factors affecting breastfeeding among women in treatment for opioid use is a complex issue with many possible directions for future research. This presentation will highlight several directions. First of all, further investigation into the decision to breastfeed among women in treatment for opioid use is needed in order to effectively promote breastfeeding among this population. Currently, most of the research seems to describe breastfeeding among drug abusing women, but not specifically opioid dependent women. Secondly, further research is needed to examine the relationship between human milk from a bottle and NAS severity. If human milk from a bottle has the same beneficial effects as breastfeeding, more women in treatment for opioid use may be able to breastfeed exclusively.

Interventions and Programs that Promote Breastfeeding

While the cultural stigma of opioid abuse prevents many women from seeking prenatal care, pregnancy can also serve as motivation for some to seek help for their addictions (Ballard, 2002). These women typically undergo methadone or buprenorphine maintenance therapies to manage their drug addictions during pregnancy. Research has shown that these treatments decrease the mother's use of illicit drugs and other opiates, while also lowering maternal morbidity and mortality rates (Pritham, Paul, & Hayes, 2012). Opiate maintenance therapies increase the mother's adherence to prenatal care and advice, furthermore protecting the fetus by promoting fetal stability and growth (Pritham et al., 2012; Pritham, 2013). Methadone Maintenance Therapies (MMT) and Buprenorphine Maintenance Therapies are associated with factors that are beneficial to the mother and the infant. Therefore, opioid-maintenance therapies are not deemed contraindications to breastfeeding (Wong, Ordean, & Kahan, 2011).

For infants of opioid-dependent mothers in treatment, breast-feeding serves as an appropriate treatment for managing infant withdrawal and has been associated with a decreased need for treatment of NAS (Welle-Strand et al., 2013). Breastfeeding also promotes responsibility and structure for the mother, raising the mother's self-esteem (Williams, 1985). Although breastfeeding is beneficial for this population of women, the Academy of Breastfeeding and Medicine suggests a criterion be used when determining which of these women should be encouraged to breastfeed (ABM Clinical Protocol #21, 2009). Specific breastfeeding policies for chemically dependent mothers vary between hospital settings. Though policies may be added that make breastfeeding eligibility requirements contingent upon the mother's substance use in the third trimester, or promote increased urine surveillance of these women in MMT. In the case of most hospital policies, if a women tests positive for any substance other than methadone, she will not be recommended to breastfeed (Williams, 1985).

Some of the challenges of promoting breastfeeding among this group of mothers stem from the lack of evidence-based guidelines for chemically dependent women wishing to breastfeed. Without the continuity of guidelines and policies, medical professionals may be inadequately trained on how to manage breastfeeding for opioid-addicted women in MMT (Schanler, O'Connor, & Lawrence, 1999). However, there are interventions that are beneficial for the promotion of breastfeeding. For healthy women, peer support is advantageous to breastfeeding. These peer supporters serve breastfeeding moms as role models familiar with the challenges of breastfeeding. Peer support/counseling increases breastfeeding duration and exclusivity (Demitras, 2012; Wambach et al., 2005). An informal, personalized approach to prenatal health education, as well as physician encouragement, increases breastfeeding initiation among women of low income and low education (Demitras, 2012; Dyson, McCormick, & Renfrew, 2005; Wambach et al., 2005). In addition, breastfeeding initiation and duration rates among low income women have increased through participation in lactation programs that include motivational videos during prenatal care and a one year of follow-up with a lactation consultant (Demitras, 2012).

Policies regarding breastfeeding and opiate-dependent mothers are not consistent across hospitals. However, several breastfeeding interventions in hospitals look promising for this population of women (Pritham, 2013). One such intervention is rooming-in. Infants of chemically dependent mothers are most at risk for attachment and abandonment issues. The early postpartum separation of the opioid-addicted mother and infant can be detrimental to the mother-infant bond. The rooming-in intervention allows the infant and the mother to remain in the same room, which as a result, increases breastfeeding rates during the hospital stay (Abrahams et al., 2007; Pritham et al., 2012). Another successful intervention is early postpartum skin-to-skin contact between the drug-dependent mother and infant. This intervention increases infant awareness, has positive effects on maternal feelings, and also increases breastfeeding initiation (Pritham, 2013). Integrated medical and behavioral program interventions are also advantageous due to the frequency of psychiatric issues among women in treatment for opioid use. In these programs, mothers are encouraged to bring their infants to sessions facilitated by psychologists. Resident physicians, nurse practitioners, and lactation consultants also attend the group. Mothers receive patient education on the risks and symptoms of NAS, and breastfeeding is modeled by the health professionals. Integrated programs have demonstrated an increase in breastfeeding initiation and duration rates among participants (O'Connor, Collett, William, & O'Brien, 2013).

As research has shown, breastfeeding is beneficial for the chemically dependent mother and her infant. For this reason, further exploration of techniques and interventions used to increase breastfeeding among this population is needed. Increasing the quality of professional training and education among health professionals so that they are fully equipped to understand and manage such a complex group of women is another vital step. The collaboration between health professionals and the community is also important, since both are an integral part of pre- and post-natal care. Future research should analyze the continuity of support messages from the community and the health professionals who care for these women. These preliminary results are promising medical strides made to help opioid-addicted women and their infants through breastfeeding. However, future work is necessary.

References

ABM clinical protocol #21: Guidelines for breastfeeding and the drug-dependent woman. (2009). *Breastfeeding Medicine, 4*(4), 225-228.

Abdel-Latif, M. E., Pinner, J., Clews, S., Cooke, F., Lui, K., & Oei, J. (2006). Effects of breast milk on the severity and outcomes of neonatal abstinence syndrome among infants of drug-dependent mothers. *Pediatrics, 117*(6), e1163-e1169.

Abrahams, R. R., Kelly, S. A., Payne, S., Thiessen, P. N., Mackintosh, J., & Janssen, P. A. (2007). Rooming-in compared with standard care for newborns of mothers using methadone or heroin. *Canadian Family Physician, 53*, 1722-1730.

Alto, W. A., & O'Connor, A. B. (2011). Management of women treated with buprenorphine during pregnancy. *American Journal of Obstetrics and Gynecology, 205*(4), 302-308.

American Academy of Pediatrics, Committee on Drugs. (1998). Neonatal drug withdrawal. *Pediatrics, 101*(6), 1079-1089.

Ballard, J. A. (2002). Treatment of neonatal abstinence syndrome with human milk containing methadone. *Journal of Perinatal and Neonatal Nursing, 15*(4), 76-85.

Backes, C. H., Backes, C. R., Gardner, D., Nankervis, C. A., Giannone, P. H., & Cordero, L. (2012). Neonatal abstinence syndrome: Transitioning methadone-treated infants from an inpatient to an outpatient setting. *Journal of Perinatology, 32*, 425-430.

Bauer, C. R., Shankaran, S., Bada, H. S., Lester, B., Wright, L. L., Krause-Steinrauf, H., & Verter, J. (2002). The maternal lifestyle study: Drug exposure during pregnancy and short-term maternal outcomes. *American Journal of Obstetrics and Gynecology, 186*(3), 487-495.

Demitras, B. (2012). Strategies to support breastfeeding: A review. *International Nursing Review, 59*, 474-481.

Dyson, L., McCormick, F. M., & Renfrew, M. J. (2005). Interventions for promoting the initiation of breastfeeding. *Cochrane Database of Systematic Reviews 2005*, (2), CD001688.

Giugliani, E. R. J., Caiaffa, W. T., Vogelhut, J., Witter, F. R., & Perman, J. A. (1994). Effects of breastfeeding support from different sources on mothers' decisions to breastfeed. *Journal of Human Lactation, 10*(3), 157-161.

Jansson, L. M., Choo, R., Velez, M. L., Harrow, C., Schroeder, J. R., Shakleya, D. M., & Huestis, M. A. (2008). Methadone maintenance and breastfeeding in the neonatal period. *Pediatrics, 121*, 106-114.

Jansson, L. M., & Velez, M. (2012). Neonatal abstinence syndrome. Current Opinion in *Pediatrics, 24*(2), 252-258.

Kandall, S. R., Albin, S., Gartner, L. M., Lee, K. S., Eidelman, A., & Lowinson, J. (1977). The narcotic dependent mother: Fetal and neonatal consequences. *Early Human Development, 1*(2), 159-169.

McCarthy, J. J., & Posey, B. L. (2000). Methadone levels in human milk. *Journal of Human Lactation, 16*, 115-120.

National Institute on Drug Abuse. (2005). Research report series - heroin abuse and addiction. Retrieved February 12, 2014, from National Institute on Drug Abuse website: http://www.drugabuse.gov/publications/research-reports/heroin-abuse-addiction

O'Connor, A. B., Collett, A., William, A. A., & O'Brien, L. M. (2013). Breastfeeding rate and the relationship between breastfeeding and neonatal abstinence syndrome in women maintained on buprenorphine during pregnancy. *Journal of Midwifery and Women's Health, 58*, 383-388.

Pritham, U. A. (2013). Breastfeeding promotion for management of neonatal abstinence syndrome. *Journal of Obstetric, Gynecologic, and Neonatal Nursing, 42*, 517-526.

Pritham, U. A., Paul, J. A., & Hayes, M. J. (2012). Opioid dependency in pregnancy and length of stay for neonatal abstinence syndrome. *Journal of Obstetric, Gynecologic, and Neonatal Nursing, 41*(2), 180-190.

Schanler, R. J., O'Connor, K. G., & Lawrence, R. A. (1999). Pediatricians' practices and attitudes regarding breastfeeding promotion. *American Academy of Pediatrics, 103*(3), 1-5.

Substance Abuse and Mental Health Services Administration. (2011, September). Results from the 2010 national survey on drug use and health: Summary of national findings. Retrieved from http://www.oas.samhsa.gov/NSDUH/2k10NSDUH/2k10Results.pdf

The American College of Obstetricians and Gynecologists; Committee on Health Care for Underserved Women and the American Society of Addiction Medicine. (2012). Opioid abuse, dependence, and addiction in pregnancy. *American Journal of Obstetrics and Gynecology, 119*(5), 1070-1076.

Wambach, K., Campbell, S. H., Gill, S. L., Dodgson, J. E., Abiona, T. C., & Heinig, M. J. (2005). Clinical lactation practice: 20 years of evidence. *Journal of Human Lactation, 21*(3), 245-258.

Welle-Strand, G. K., Skurtveit, S., Jansson, L. M., Brittelise, B., Bjarko, B., & Ravndal, E. (2013). Breastfeeding reduces the need for withdrawal treatment in opioid-exposed infants. *Acta Pedeatrica, 102*, 1060-1066.

Williams, A. (1985). When the client is pregnant: Information for counselors. *Journal of Substance Abuse Treatment, 2*, 27-35.

Wong, S., Ordean, A., & Kahan, M. (2011). Substance use in pregnancy. *Journal of Obstetrics and Gynaecology Canada, 33*(4), 367-38

Depressed and the Breast: The Intersection of Breastfeeding and Postpartum Depression

Deborah McCarter-Spaulding

It is frequently reported that there is a relationship between postpartum depression (PPD) and breastfeeding. However, the relationship remains unclear in several domains, including breastfeeding intention, initiation, duration, and pattern.

Intention: Very little is written about the relationship of a history of depression and the intent to breastfeed one's infant, even though it is well-accepted that intention to breastfeed is a predictor of breastfeeding. Bogen, Hanusa, Moses-Kolko and Wisner (2010) reported that depression during pregnancy did not predict intention to breastfeed, but receiving medication during pregnancy did predict an increased likelihood of intending to formula feed. McKee, Zayas, and Jankowski (2004) also found no relationship between depression during pregnancy and feeding intent. However, Fairlie, Gillman, and Rich-Edwards (2009) did find that prenatal depression symptoms, as well as prenatal anxiety, were associated with planning to formula feed.

Initiation: Many studies reported initiation of breastfeeding was not influenced by prenatal depression (Bogen et al., 2010; Fairlie et al., 2009; Pippins, Brawarsky, Jackson, Fuentes-Afflick, & Haas, 2006), but some did report that prenatal depression decreased breastfeeding initiation (Dennis & McQueen, 2009; Figueiredo, Canario, & Field, 2013; Hamdan & Tamin, 2012).

Duration: Many studies report that there is an association with breastfeeding and postpartum depression, with higher depression scores associated with shorter duration (Dunn, Davis, McCleary, Edwards, & Gaboury, 2006; Henderson, Evans, Straton, Priest, & Hagan, 2003; Pippins et al., 2006; Watkins, Meltzer-Brody, Zolnoun, & Stuebe, 2011). Some studies did not find an association (Bogen et al., 2010; McKee et al., 2004). Some found an association at some time points, but not others (Dennis & McQueen, 2009).

Exclusivity/Pattern: Many studies found that depression was associated with less exclusive breastfeeding at some time points (Dennis & McQueen, 2007; Gaffney, Kitsantas, Brito, & Swamidoss, 2014; Hahn-Holbrook, Haselton, Dunkel Schetter, & Glynn, 2013; Hatton et al., 2005; Henderson et al., 2003; Watkins et al., 2011). Some studies found no association between exclusivity and depression (Bogen et al., 2010).

There are many confounding variables, including the time of measurement, with the influence of depression being significant in early breastfeeding (4 to 6 weeks), but not later (8 to 12 weeks) (Dennis & McQueen, 2007; Hatton et al., 2005), or whether a mother was experiencing breastfeeding problems or pain in the early postpartum period (Watkins et al., 2011), in addition to psychosocial variables, such as the strength of the intention to breastfeed (Bogen et al., 2010) or confidence (Bogen et al., 2010; Field, Hernandez-Reif, & Fiejo, 2002).

The temporality of the relationship between PPD and breastfeeding is unclear, particularly since many of the studies are cross-sectional. Longitudinal studies have noted that depression precedes weaning (Dennis & McQueen, 2007), while others found breastfeeding to be protective (Hahn-Holbrook et al., 2013). Results varied depending on the time measured (Hatton et al., 2005), and on demographic factors (McKee et al., 2004), such as race/ethnicity and socioeconomic status.

Research is currently underway in a sample of women recruited from the maternity unit of a New Hampshire hospital, testing the effectiveness of an educational intervention on the reduction of postpartum depression symptoms. As part of this larger study, breast-feeding outcomes were measured. In this sample, prenatal anxiety and prenatal depression had a significant negative effect on the intent to breastfeed exclusively. A history of depression prior to pregnancy and current symptoms of postpartum depression, both appear to have a negative effect on exclusive breastfeeding as well as earlier weaning compared to those without depression. Further results will be available when data collection is complete.

The importance of addressing breastfeeding and maternal mental health simultaneously concerns many professional disciplines, including mental health, obstetrics, pediatrics, and lactation. In the prenatal period, current and previous history of mood disorders, as well as infant feeding intent should be considered together. Anticipatory guidance about expectations, management of breastfeeding problems, and fatigue should be provided, as well as referrals to mental health services. Medication management of depression either prenatally or postpartum must take into consideration a woman's breastfeeding goals, and the potential emotional impact on her ability to meet those goals, or manage the process of loss if she is unable to do so. Depression is likely to be influenced by the value of breastfeeding to the mother, requiring consideration of motivation, confidence, feelings of guilt, and cultural influences on feeding choice.

Lactation consultants and other obstetrical health providers must be alert to the potential co-morbidity of breastfeeding problems and postpartum depression. Management of each must involve consideration of the other, in the context of the individual family's needs, goals, and resources. Assessment for postpartum depression symptoms may be a skill needed by lactation consultants and pediatric providers, just as lactation expertise is an essential resource for pediatric and obstetric providers. Mental health providers who are aware of the meaning of breastfeeding to mothers, as well as the health benefits of and challenges inherent in the experience will be able to provide treatment and recommendations which more holistically meet the needs of breastfeeding women and babies. It is clear that there is no single recommendation for all mothers/families. Management of both breastfeeding and depression is significant to the health and well-being of mothers, newborns, and families. Research, education, and practice must reflect knowledge of the interaction between maternal mood disorders and lactation in order to provide appropriate, compassionate, and evidence-based care.

References

Bogen, D. L., Hanusa, B. H., Moses-Kolko, E., & Wisner, K. L. (2010). Are maternal depression or symptom severity associated with breastfeeding intention or outcomes? *The Journal of Clinical Psychiatry, 71*(8), 1069-1078. doi: 10.4088/JCP.09m05383blu

Dennis, C.-L., & McQueen, K. (2007). Does maternal postpartum depressive symptomatology influence infant feeding outcomes? *Acta Paediatrica (Oslo, Norway: 1992), 96*(4), 590-594.

Dennis, C.-L., & McQueen, K. (2009). The relationship between infant-feeding outcomes and postpartum depression: A qualitative systematic review. *Pediatrics, 123*(4), e736-e751. doi: 10.1542/peds.2008-1629

Dunn, S., Davis, B., McCleary, L., Edwards, N., & Gaboury, I. (2006). The relationship between vulnerability factors and breastfeeding outcome. *JOGNN: Journal of Obstetric, Gynecologic & Neonatal Nursing, 35*, 87-97. doi: 10.1111/J.1552-6909.2006.00005.x

Fairlie, T. G., Gillman, M. W., & Rich-Edwards, J. (2009). High pregnancy-related anxiety and prenatal depressive symptoms as predictors of intention to breastfeed and breastfeeding initiation. *Journal of Women's Health (2002), 18*(7), 945-953. doi: 10.1089/jwh.2008.0998

Field, T., Hernandez-Reif, M., & Fiejo, L. (2002). Breastfeeding in depressed mother-infant dyads. *Early Child Development and Care, 172*, 539-545. doi: 10.1080/0300443022000046787

Figueiredo, B., Canario, C., & Field, T. (2013). Breastfeeding is negatively affected by prenatal depression and reduces postpartum depression. *Psychological Medicine, 1-10.*

Gaffney, K. F., Kitsantas, P., Brito, A., & Swamidoss, C. S. S. (2014). Postpartum depression, infant feeding practices, and infant weight gain at six months of age. *Journal of Pediatric Health Care: Official Publication of National Association of Pediatric Nurse Associates & Practitioners, 28*(1), 43-50. doi: dx.doi.org/10.1016/j.pedhc.2012.10.005

Hahn-Holbrook, J., Haselton, M. G., Dunkel Schetter, C., & Glynn, L. M. (2013). Does breastfeeding offer protection against maternal depressive symptomatology?: A prospective study from pregnancy to 2 years after birth. *Archives of Women's Mental Health, 16*(5), 411-422. doi: 10.1007/s00737-013-0348-9

Hamdan, A., & Tamin, H. (2012). The relationship between postpartum depression and breastfeeding. *International Journal of Psychiatry in Medicine, 43*(3), 243-259. doi: 10.2190/PM.43.3.d

Hatton, D. C., Harrison-Hohner, J., Coste, S., Dorato, V., Curet, L. B., & McCarron, D. A. (2005). Symptoms of postpartum depression and breastfeeding. *Journal of Human Lactation, 21*(4), 444-449. doi: 10.1177/0890334405280947

Henderson, J. J., Evans, S. F., Straton, J. A. Y., Priest, S. R., & Hagan, R. (2003). Impact of postnatal depression on breastfeeding duration. *Birth: Issues in Perinatal Care, 30*(3), 175-180.

McKee, M. D., Zayas, L. H., & Jankowski, K. R. B. (2004). Breastfeeding intention and practice in an urban minority population: Relationship to maternal depressive symptoms and mother-infant closeness. *Journal of Reproductive & Infant Psychology, 22*(3), 167-181. doi: 10.1080/02646830410001723751

Pippins, J. R., Brawarsky, P., Jackson, R. A., Fuentes-Afflick, E., & Haas, J. S. (2006). Association of breastfeeding with maternal depressive symptoms. *Journal of Women's Health, 15*(6), 754-762.

Watkins, S., Meltzer-Brody, S., Zolnoun, D., & Stuebe, A. (2011). Early breastfeeding experiences and postpartum depression. *Obstetrics & Gynecology, 118*(2 Pt 1), 214-221. doi: http://dx.doi.org/10.1097/AOG.0b013e3182260a2d

An Adaptive Leadership Perspective on the Discrepancy Between Planned and Reported Home Infant Sleep Locations

Kristin P. Tully, Diane Holditch-Davis, and Debra Brandon

Despite medical recommendations against parent-infant bedsharing in the U.S. (American Academy of Pediatrics, 2011), the prevalence of at least occasional bedsharing among American families is estimated to be between 42% to 7% (Hauck, Signore, Fein, & Raju, 2008; Lahr, Rosenberg, & Lapidus, 2005; Willinger, Ko, Hoffman, Kessler, & Corwin, 2003). Practical, evidence-based support is necessary to optimize infant sleep environments because bedsharing has been positively associated with breastfeeding (Ball, 2003; Blair, Heron, & Fleming, 2010; Huang et al., 2013; Santos, Mota, Matijasevich, Barros, & Barros, 2009) and with Sudden Infant Death Syndrome (SIDS; Carpenter et al., 2013). Nighttime arrangements are a personal issue for families. However, physician guidelines do not include recommendations about the need to dialogue with families about infant sleep locations (American Academy of Pediatrics, 2011).

Coproduced solutions between health care professionals and families may be effective for promoting healthful infant sleep environments. In particular, adaptive leadership is the practice of facilitating learning and behavior change to optimize well-being over time

(Thygeson, Morrissey, & Ulstad, 2010). This framework encourages ongoing teamwork to create achievable strategies. Adaptive challenges are those that involve learning and trade-offs (Thygeson et al., 2010), which would include changing a parental behavior, such as infant sleep locations, as described by Ball and Volpe (2013). However, the factors that contribute to decisions about infant-sleep locations in the context of individual families' needs and preferences are currently unclear.

This study investigated maternal report of planned and practiced home infant-sleep locations over the first postpartum month. The objective was to better understand how nocturnal infant feeding and other nighttime needs affect decisions about infant sleep in the home. The study compared women who gave birth to late preterm infants (34 0/7 to 36 6/7 gestational weeks) with those who gave birth at term ($\geq$ 37 0/7 gestational weeks) to determine the challenges over the first postpartum month. Although previous research found that American infants born prematurely were more likely to bedshare than term infants (Colson et al., 2013), how late preterm birth might affect infant sleep locations in the home is unknown. Therefore, the purpose of this study was to describe parent-infant sleep plans and reported practices of the late preterm and term dyads.

Method

This observational multi-method study was conducted from 2010 to 2012.

Participants

Mothers and their infants were recruited from a regional referral birthing center of a southeastern academic medical center with approximately 3,300 births per year. Term participants were matched to late preterm participants on maternal race/ethnicity and mode of delivery.

Mothers were excluded from the larger study (Brandon et al., 2011). If they did not have custody of the infant, the mother's situation would have affected her ability to participate (age less than 18; history of HIV, psychosis, or bipolar disease; or non-English speaking). Infants were singletons and their health was not an inclusion or exclusion criterion.

Participants for this analysis were asked specific questions about sleep locations, which were added in the middle of the larger study. Fifty-six women provided hospital interview data (26 late preterm and 30 term), and 45 of these participants (22 late preterm and 23 term) provided telephone interview data at one month postpartum. Participant demographics by late preterm and term status are provided in Table 1.

Table 1

Participant Demographics, by Late Preterm and Term Groups

	Late Preterm n=26	Term n=30
	Mean (SD) or % (n)	Mean (SD) or % (n)
Maternal race and ethnicity:		
% White non-Hispanic	56.0 (14)	50.0 (15)
% Black non-Hispanic	32.0 (8)	33.3 (10)
% Hispanic and Other	12.0 (3)	16.7 (5)
% Married	69.2 (18)	43.3 (13)
% Public assistance	38.5 (10)	43.4 (13)
% First-time mother*	11.5 (3)	40.0 (12)
Maternal age in years*	31.0 (6.5)	26.8 (5.0)
% Had any pregnancy complications	61.5 (16)	36.7 (11)
Gestational age in weeks***	35.9 (.8)	40.0 (.9)
Infant sex: % female	57.7 (15)	43.3 (13)
% Cesarean birth	46.2 (12)	36.7 (11)

Birthweight in grams	2693.3 (470.2)	3408.8 (446.7)
Apgar at 1 minute	7.6 (2.1)	8.0 (1.6)
Apgar at 5 minutes*	8.7 (.7)	9.0 (.3)
% Only in well baby nursery*	73.1 (19)	93.3 (28)
Length of hospital stay in days*	4.9 (5.5)	2.3 (.7)
% Provided human milk:		
Postpartum hospitalization	76.9 (20)	93.3 (28)
One month postpartum	65.2 (15)	74.1 (20)

Note. Between-group mean differences on continuous variables were tested using *t*-tests, except for length of infant hospital stay that was tested with a non-parametric Wilcoxon Two Sample Test due to non-normal distribution. Between-group differences in proportions were tested using Cochran-Mantel-Haenzel, chi-square, or the Fisher's Exact Test, as appropriate.

* $p<.05$ for group differences; ***$p<.0001$

Measures

Maternal and Infant Characteristics: Demographic information was reported by the mother. Infant medical records were reviewed after enrollment and following hospital discharge to obtain data on obstetric history and medical course.

Semi-Structured Interviews: The hospital interview focused on the mother's childbirth story and her infant's care. The interview began with a global statement asking the mother to tell her story about how she "came to deliver." Probes were asked to elicit greater detail when needed and to fill in predetermined areas not covered such as "what are you currently feeding your baby" and "where do you plan for your infant to sleep at home?" After a mother responded with her intended infant sleep location, she was asked if she "also planned to bedshare." At one month postpartum, the interviews explored how things had been going with the mother and her infant since the previous interview. Once the mother told her story, probes were used to cover predetermined topics, which included feeding and sleep practices. After a mother responded to "where is your baby currently sleeping a night," she was asked if she had "also slept with the baby in bed with [her]."

Procedure

Following Institutional Review Board approval, a research team member confirmed potential eligibility and the appropriateness of potential participation with the nursing staff. Mothers were approached on the postnatal unit, the day after childbirth or later. Immediately after a mother provided written informed consent to participate in the study or at a time more convenient to the mother, the demographics form was administered and the semi-structured interview was conducted. Data was obtained while the mother-infant dyads were in the hospital at enrollment and discharge, and at home at 1 month postpartum. Participant responses were audio recorded, transcribed, and then checked for accuracy.

Analysis

The transcripts were read in their entirety to get a sense of the mother's story as a whole. Interviews were then read again to derive codes and their definitions (Miles, Huberman, & Saldana, 2013). Next, the codes were refined and then grouped into meaningful themes (Patton, 2001).

The responses were entered into a matrix format by theme for ease of comparison. Codes derived from research questions, such as "what factors influenced where your baby currently sleeps at night," as well as refinements of the core issues that emerged, such as "not bedsharing due to fear for infant safety," which the authors identified through an iterative process. Between-group mean differences on continuous demographic variables were examined using t-tests. Between-group differences in proportions of demographic variables, maternal milk provision, and infant-sleep locations were tested using Cochran-Mantel-Haenzel, chi-square, or the Fisher's Exact Test, as appropriate.

Results

A few participants from both the late preterm and term groups planned to bedshare. The factor most often influencing this decision was maternal convenience for nighttime infant monitoring. The other reasons were facilitating infant sleep, maternal reassurance of infant well-being, and maternal preference.

Women in both groups said that they planned not to bedshare at home due to fear for infant safety. One mother said she needed her infant "in a container" at night because she was "too scared" that she might otherwise "throw her across the room" or "smash her." Further, the idea of bedsharing becoming an undesirable habit and/or spoiling the baby was present in both the late preterm and term groups.

Significantly more women reported that they bedshared with their infant during the first postpartum month (21 of 44, 47.7%) than said that they had planned to do so (6 of 56, 10.7%), $X^2=15.3$, $df=1$, $p<.0001$. Late preterm and term groups did not differ in unplanned bedsharing. All mothers who planned on bedsharing reported doing so. The reasons offered for bedsharing were similar between the late preterm and term groups, with nighttime infant fussiness being the primary factor. Other reasons for bedsharing were maternal preference/

emotional closeness, reassurance of infant well-being, convenience with nighttime feeds, early morning rest, daytime naps, and lack of a bassinet (term mother). One of the mothers who bedshared did so because she was told the baby (born late preterm) had to be upright for a prolonged period after feeding. This positioning was accomplished by having the baby propped on pillows in the adult bed alongside the mother who returned to sleep.

Among those who did not bedshare, some mothers added that they did not do so because they were afraid for infant safety. One of the term mothers who did not bedshare routinely co-slept with her infant on a recliner. She would feed the baby in the reclining armchair in the living room at night, fall asleep, and then wake up for the next feed there.

Discussion

This study followed late preterm and term infants and their mothers from the postpartum hospitalization to the first postpartum month. Some mothers' understanding of bedsharing as inappropriate conflicted with their needs for nighttime proximity to infants. Mothers were close to their infants out of preference, for convenience in assessing the babies' well-being, and for ease of tending to them. Professional guidance that works with mothers and acknowledges their constraints around infant sleep locations and provides evidence-based guidance on potential hazards may help in enabling both safe infant environments and maternal rest.

The need for individualized parent sleep guidance, as endorsed by Fetherston and Leach (2012), was highlighted in our example of a mother who bedshared with a late preterm infant propped on pillows. She did this to comply with the pediatrician's advice to position the baby upright for an extended period after feedings, and the need to achieve this arrangement in a way that permitted maternal sleep.

Maternal decision making for high-needs infants may be impaired by fatigue from managing health challenges over time.

Maternal convenience in nighttime infant monitoring was the primary reason for mothers intending to bedshare. In order to have the safest infant sleep environments possible, families may benefit from health care providers facilitating non-judgmental discussions about nighttime dynamics (e.g., United Nations Children's Fund UK, 2011). Many more families said that they bedshared during the first post-partum month than planned to do so. A similar pattern was also found by Stremler and colleagues (2013). The discrepancy we found between bedsharing plans and practice suggests that maternal expectations for nighttime parenting and infant sleep did not match their experiences.

Fear for infant safety was commonly discussed among participants who avoided bedsharing, which may stem from U.S. public education campaigns that focus on the hazards of bedsharing (e.g., http://city.milwaukee.gov/Safe-Sleep-Campaign). However, observational studies with healthy breastfeeding dyads suggest these mother-infant pairs largely sleep and wake in synchrony (McKenna, Ball, & Gettler, 2007), face each other, and maintain close proximity for most of the night and that these mothers adopt a protective sleep position around their sleeping infants (Baddock, Galland, Taylor, & Bolton, 2007; Ball, 2006). Bottle feeding mothers, on the other hand, have been observed sleeping with infants more "like an adult' in the bed, with the babies positioned higher than breast level, and the mothers turned away from the infants (Ball, 2006). Further, any infant sleep location can become hazardous, such as with the use of inappropriate bedding materials or impaired caregivers (Volpe, Ball, & McKenna, 2013).

Nighttime infant feedings are often accompanied by mother-infant sleep in the feeding locations, including beds, sofas, and recliners (Kendall-Tackett, Cong, & Hale, 2010). Kendall-Tackett and colleagues (2010) found that mothers who slept with their infants in feeding locations tended to have high incomes and more education. These researchers suggest that this otherwise "low-risk" group engaged in high-risk behavior in an attempt to avoid bedsharing, which is consistent with our finding about the mother who co-slept with her infant on a recliner. Conversations among health care providers and families may advance understanding of infant sleep location recommendations away from the "letter of the law" to the "spirit."

Although our sample was diverse and reflective of the community from which it was drawn, it was limited by the exclusion of families with multiple births and of non-English speaking mothers. The dynamics of nighttime parenting with infants for a multiple birth set likely differs from the care of singletons. Also, the culture of parenting may vary between English and non-English speaking Hispanic mothers.

Our study grouped participants by late preterm and term childbirth status to focus on the role of infant medical needs and maternal perinatal experiences on home sleep location decisions. The within group differences we found in maternal attitudes regarding infant sleep location likely reflect maternal demographics. Strengths of this study include the prospective design, matching late preterm and term participants on maternal race, ethnicity, and childbirth mode, and probing for whether mothers' sleep plans and practice included bedsharing.

Conclusions

The discrepancy between planned and reported home infant sleep locations indicates that mothers' expectations are not consistent with their needs. Both the late preterm and term groups experienced variability in their home infant sleep locations, and women within the groups had differing feelings about bedsharing. Professional dialogues with parents that acknowledge the adaptive challenges associated with infant sleep may be more attuned to the realities of family preferences and constraints, thereby promoting safe infant sleep environments and breastfeeding.

References

American Academy of Pediatrics [AAP]. (2011). SIDS and other sleep-related infant deaths: Expansion of recommendations for a safe infant sleeping environment. *Pediatrics, 128*(5), 1030-1038. doi: 10.1542/peds.2011-2284.

Baddock, S. A., Galland, B. C., Taylor, B. J., & Bolton, D. P. G. (2007). Sleeping arrangements and behavior of bed-sharing families in the home setting. *Pediatrics, 119*(1), e200-e207. doi: 10.1542/peds.2006-0744

Ball, H. L. (2003). Breastfeeding, bed-sharing and infant sleep. *Birth, 30*(3), 181-188. doi: 10.1046/j.1523-536X.2003.00243.x

Ball, H. L. (2006). Parent-infant bed-sharing behavior: Effects of feeding type and presence of father. *Human Nature, 17*(3), 301-318.

Ball, H. L., & Volpe, L. E. (2013). Sudden Infant Death Syndrome (SIDS) risk reduction and infant sleep location – Moving the discussion forward. *Social Science & Medicine, 79*, 84-91. doi:10.1016/j.socscimed.2012.03.025

Blair, P. S., Heron, J., & Fleming, P. J. (2010). Relationship between bed sharing and breastfeeding: Longitudinal, population-based analysis. *Pediatrics, 126*(5), e1119-e1126. doi: 10.1542/peds.2010-1277

Brandon, D. H., Tully, K. P., Silva, S., Thompson, J., Malcolm, W., Murtha, A., Turner, B., & Holditch-Davis, D. (2011). Emotional responses of mothers of late-preterm and term infants. *Journal of Obstetric, Gynecologic, & Neonatal Nursing, 40*(6), 719-731. doi: 10.1111/j.1552-6909.2011.01290.x

Carpenter, R., McGarvey, C., Mitchell, E. A., Tappin, D. M., Vennemann, M. M., Smuk, M., & Carpenter, J. R. (2013). Bed sharing when parents do not smoke: Is there a risk of SIDS? An individual level analysis of five major case-control studies. *BMJ Open, 3*, e002299. doi: 10.1136/bmjopen-2012-002299.

Colson, E. R., Willinger, M., Rybin, D., Heeren, T., Smith, L. A., Lister, G., & Corwin, M. J. (2013). Trends and factors associated with infant bed sharing, 1993-2010: The National Infant Sleep Position Study. *JAMA Pediatrics, 167*(11), 1032-1037. doi: 10.1001/jamapediatrics.2013.2560.

Fetherston, C. M., & Leach, J. S. (2012). Analysis of the ethical issues in the breastfeeding and bedsharing debate. *Breastfeeding Review, 20*(3), 7-17.

Hauck, F. R., Signore, C., Fein, S. B., & Raju, T. N. K. (2008). Infant sleeping arrangements and practices during the first year of life. *Pediatrics, 122*(S2), S113-S120. doi: 10.1542/peds.2008-1315o

Huang, Y., Hauck, F. R., Signore, C., Yu, A., Raju, T. N. K., Huang, T. T.-K., & Fein, S. B. (2013). Influence of bedsharing activity on breastfeeding duration among US mothers. *JAMA Pediatrics, 167*(11), 1038-1044. doi:10.1001/jamapediatrics.2013.2632

Kendall-Tackett, K., Cong, Z., & Hale, T. W. (2010). Mother-infant sleep locations and nighttime feeding behavior. *Clinical Lactation, 1*(1), 27-31.

Lahr, M. B., Rosenberg, K. D., & Lapidus, J. A. (2005). Bedsharing and maternal smoking in a population-based survey of new mothers. *Pediatrics, 116*(4), e530-e542. doi: 10.1542/peds.2005-0354

McKenna, J. J., Ball, H. L., & Gettler, L. T. (2007). Mother-infant cosleeping, breastfeeding and sudden infant death syndrome: What biological anthropology has discovered about normal infant sleep and pediatric sleep medicine. *American Journal of Physical Anthropology, Supp 145*, 133-161. doi: 10.1002/ajpa

Miles, M.B., Huberman, A.M., & Saldana, J. (2013). *Qualitative data analysis: A methods sourcebook, 3ʳᵈ Ed.* Newbury Park, CA: Sage.

Patton, M.Q. (2001). *Qualitative research & evaluation methods, 3ʳᵈ Ed.* Newbury Park, CA: Sage.

Santos, I. S., Mota, D. M., Matijasevich, A., Barros, A. J. D., & Barros, F. C. F. (2009). Bed-sharing at 3 months and breast-feeding at 1 year in southern Brazil. *The Journal of Pediatrics, 155*(4), 505-509. doi: 10.1016/j.jpeds.2009.04.037

Stremler, R., Hodnett, E., Kenton, L., Lee, K., Macfarlane, J., Weiss, S., Weston, J., & Willan, A. (2013). Infant sleep location: Bed sharing, room sharing and solitary sleeping at 6 and 12 weeks postpartum. *The Open Sleep Journal, 6(*Suppl 1: M10), 77-86.

Thygeson, M., Morrissey, L., & Ulstad, V. (2010). Adaptive leadership and the practice of medicine: A complexity-based approach reframing the doctor-patient relationship. *Journal of Evaluation of Clinical Practice, 16*(5), 1009-1015.

United Nations Children's Fund [UNICEF] UK. (2011). *Caring for your baby at night.* Retrieved from http://www.unicef.org.uk/Documents/Baby_Friendly/Leaflets/caringatnight_web.pdf

Volpe, L. E., Ball, H. L., & McKenna, J. J. (2013). Nighttime parenting strategies and sleep-related risks to infants. *Social Science & Medicine, 79*, 92-100. http://dx.doi.org/10.1016/j.socscimed.2012.05.043

Willinger, M., Ko, C. W., Hoffman, H. J., Kessler, R. C., & Corwin, M. J. (2003). Trends in infant bed sharing in the United States, 1993-2000: the National Infant Sleep Position study. *Archives of Pediatrics & Adolescent Medicine, 157*(1), 43-49. doi:10.1001/archpedi.157.1.43

CHAPTER 22

Breastfeeding and Family Planning: Current Thinking and Potential Impact on Women

Miriam Labbok

B reastfeeding has long been recognized as having an impact on fertility return postpartum. This "old wives' tale" has now been confirmed by both demographic and biological research. The delay in the return of fertility is mediated by the pattern of breastfeeding. More intensive patterns of breastfeeding are associated, in general, with a longer inter-pregnancy interval.

It was not until 1988 that there was consideration of a method that might allow the individual to know when her fertility might return postpartum. At that time, a group of researchers gathered in Bellagio Rockefeller Conference Center to consider how ongoing research on the issue might inform the development of a new method of family planning. This group, organized and led by Dr. Kathy Kennedy at Family Health International at that time, analyzed existing data and found that three criteria would define the period of infertility: amenorrhea, full breastfeeding, and 6 months postpartum (timing based on the recognition that complementary feeding should start at that time).

These findings were later incorporated into an algorithm, and this algorithm/method was named Lactational Amenorrhea Method (LAM) during a subsequent meeting held at Georgetown University. This method then underwent clinical trial, and was found to be highly efficacious, comparable to the use of other modern contraceptives. The initial trials, sponsored by Institute for Reproductive Health at Georgetown, Family Health International, WHO, South-to-South Foundation, were held in more than 10 countries around the world. These trials found pregnancy rates varying from 0.5% to 2% by 6-month life table.

Given this, we are tempted to ask, "If LAM's so darn good, why ain't it famous?" In fact, very few women worldwide have been informed about this freely available method of family planning (FP). A review commissioned by IRH at Georgetown found that family planning programs are "distrustful" of non-commodity-based, woman-controlled, and behavior-based methods. This limited interest among the FP community is compounded by the fact that many child survival programs hesitate to support family planning. Nonetheless, the method was officially accepted in at least 40 countries, and by the World Health Organization, as a highly efficacious, albeit short-lived, method for the postpartum period.

The duration of possible use and method flexibility were also considered by examining multiple studies at a meeting referred to as Bellagio II (Kennedy, Labbok, & Van Look, 1996). At this meeting, it was concluded that the method was quite flexible, allowing for some supplementary feeding, and could be used well beyond 6 months, if the pattern of frequent breastfeeding was maintained while complementary foods were added after a breastfeed. In addition, this meeting defined menses return for LAM use as either two days of consecutive bleeding, or bleeding that the mother recognizes as menses.

The remaining issues have continued to be increasing uptake by family-planning program decision-makers, and increasing uptake by child survival program decision-makers, since breastfeeding remains a significant contributor to both global birthspacing and child survival rates. Without considering LAM, the family planning community has proceeded to introduce hormonal methods during breastfeeding with minimal consideration of the impact on both establishment of breastfeeding, or the possible long-term impact on the child of early exposure to exogenous hormones. There are frequent clinical reports of significantly diminished ability to breastfeed occurring rapidly, following introduction of hormonal contraception, with onset of diminished milk production within day(s), and difficulty, and at times impossibility, of re-establishing breastfeeding. These hormones can act by causing disruptions of the mammary – hypothalamic-pituitary-ovarian axis impacting breastfeeding, or may influence the establishment of breastfeeding by changing sensitivity of the areola or filling receptor sites, and may have subtle impacts on milk composition. As this has not been carefully studied, there may be additional issues that have not yet been raised.

Both WHO and CDC consider each method and the ranking of safety of its use during breastfeeding, rather than considering that women breastfeed, then discussing the safest methods to be used. Logically, it is best for the mother/baby to use non-hormonal methods during breastfeeding, and if a hormonal method is to be used, to start with a progestin-only pill after at least 6 weeks to assess impact on milk supply. The pill would allow rapid reversal if there were a negative impact. However, the Medical Eligibility Criteria examine the pros and cons for each method during breastfeeding, rather than starting with what is best for the breastfeeding mother. Therefore, all methods are considered.

In the U.S., there is a high level of use of immediate postpartum depot medroxyprogesterone acetate (DMPA, Depo-Provera™), anecdotally, predominantly among women of color and/or low-wealth populations. There are no studies at this time that have fully assessed immediate postpartum use of DMPA and its impact on breastfeeding, or its long-term potential impact on the child. Logically, it would be wise to use a different method until these studies are done. Minimally, the woman's informed consent should be documented. However, to the best of my knowledge, neither hesitancy to use the method, nor documentation of informed consent, are current practices in the U.S.

The Medical Eligibility Criteria (MEC), used by both WHO and CDC, are presented as four categories, and as a simplified two-category system, as presented here. Where a doctor or nurse is not available to make clinical judgments, the two-categories system may be considered, as shown in this table. A second table compares the WHO decisions to the CDC decision. Clearly, the WHO experts are more cautious with acceptance of methods that may disrupt breastfeeding. In sum, WHO's MEC Recommendations have been modified by CDC without, in this author's opinion, adequately balancing risks or considering alternatives. They do not address the potential health risks to mother and child of *diminished breastfeeding* in the early months postpartum, but rather prioritize preventing another pregnancy, with minimal regard to subsequent health. While it is true that an unplanned pregnancy carries a great deal of risk for both mother and child, the risks of not breastfeeding should also be considered.

Medical Eligibility Criteria (MEC) and Simplified Two Category System			WHO vs. CDC Medical Eligibility Criteria	
Where a doctor or nurse is not available to make clinical judgments, the 4-categories can be simplified into 2-categories system as shown in this table:			**WHO**	**CDC - July 2011 MMWR**
WHO Category	**With Clinical Judgment**	**With Limited Clinical Judgement**	• Combined:	❖ Combined:
1	Use the method in any circumstances	Use the method	– 4: 0-6 wks – 3: 6 wks - 6 m 2: >6 m	▶ 4: 0-3 wks ▶ 3: 3-6 wks ▶ 2: >6 wks
2	Generally use the method	Use the method	• Progestin only – 3: 0-6 wks – 1: 6 wks- 6 m 1: >6 m	❖ Progestin only ▶ 2: 0-4 wks ▶ 1: >4 wks
3	Use of the method not usually recommended unless other, more appropriate methods are not available or acceptable	Do not use the method	• LNG-IUD – 3: <48hrs – 3: 48hrs- 4 wks 1: >4 wks	❖ LNG-IUD ▶ 2: < 10 min ▶ 2: 10 m – 4 wks ▶ 1: >4 wks
4	Method not to be used	Do not use the method	• Cu-IUD – 1: <48hrs – 3: 48 hrs-4wks 1: > 4wks	❖ Cu-IUD ▶ 1: <10 min ▶ 2: 10 m – 4wks ▶ 1: > 4 wks

For many years, those who wish to support all health considerations for the mother and child have offered the First Choice Methods for use during breastfeeding, to include LAM, NFP, Barriers, IUDs, and Second Choice Methods to be the progestin-only methods, starting after 6 weeks postpartum, when lactation is well-established. The Third Choice, which should rarely be considered, and used only when the child is mostly consuming other foods, would be the combined hormonal methods.

We know that WHO is reconsidering its MEC decisions later this year. It will be of great interest to see if they follow the lead of CDC, and increase acceptability of hormonal methods during breastfeeding [Post meeting note: WHO did not relax its criteria at that meeting]. The mother herself should be front and center in any, and all, decisions about what contraceptive approach she will use. I hope this paper might provoke discussion and increase the acceptance of the mother as an informed participant in any decision concerning what drugs she is given during breastfeeding, or at any other time.

References

Centers for Disease Control and Prevention (CDC). (2010). *United States Medical Eligibility Criteria (US MEC) for contraceptive use.* Retrieved from http://www.cdc.gov/reproductivehealth/UnintendedPregnancy/USMEC.htm

Kennedy, K., Labbok, M., & Van Look, P. (1996, July). Amenorrhea method for family planning. *International Journal of Gynaecology & Obstetrics, 54*(1), 55-57.

Labbok, M. H., Perez, A., Valdes, V., Sevilla, F., Wade, K., Laukaran, V. H., Cooney, K. A., Coly, S., Sanders, C., & Queenan, J.T. (1994). The Lactational Amenorrhea Method (LAM): A postpartum introductory family planning method with policy and program implications. *Advances in Contraception, 10*, 93-109.

Labbok, M. (2008). *Global. Library of women's medicine* DOI 10.3843/GLOWM.10397 Retrieved from http://www.glowm.com/section_view/item/396

World Health Organization (WHO). *Medical eligibility criteria for contraceptive use, 4th Ed..* Retrieved from http://www.who.int/reproductivehealth/publications/family_planning/9789241563888/en/

Section IIIb

Providers of Breastfeeding Support

Breastfeeding and Health Care Personnel: Breastfeeding Peer Counselors in the NICU

Beverly Rossman

Becoming a mother, or the incorporation of motherhood into a woman's concept of herself and her perceived confidence in being a mother, is often altered unexpectedly and significantly when a woman gives birth to a very premature infant. The distress that accompanies an unanticipated, very preterm birth often compromises, or delays, the development of the maternal role, and is associated with depressive symptoms, anxiety, and psychological distress. After a premature birth, the mother seeks information about her infant's health status and what she can do to optimize her infant's outcome. Whereas milk from the infant's own mother is critical to reduce the risk of specific morbidities in premature infants during, and after, the NICU hospitalization, it has also long been seen as the "one thing that only the mother can do." Researchers have reported that the provision of milk is a unique maternal activity that provides mothers with a sense of purpose and worth, and helps them feel a connection and bond with their infants.

Although the benefits of human milk are well-documented, mothers of very premature infants encounter numerous barriers and challenges to the initiation and maintenance of lactation that are not experienced by mothers of healthy term infants including pumping factors, such as breast pump type and pumping frequency, maternal health factors linked to lower lactation success that are frequently present in mothers of very premature infants, dislike of using the breast pump, and the lifestyle inconveniences required to maintain milk volume, and stress and anxiety related to uncertainties about their infants' compromised health status (Callen & Pinelli, 2005; Cregan, De Mello, Kershaw, McDougall, & Hartmann, 2002; Hill, Aldag, Chatterton, & Zinaman, 2005a; Hill, Aldag, Chatterton, & Zinaman, 2005b; Lessen & Crivelli-Kovach, 2007; Meier, Engstrom, Patel, Jegier, & Bruns, 2010; Rossman, Kratovil, Greene, Engstrom, & Meier, 2013). Lactation care for these mothers, who are often breast pump-dependent for weeks or months, requires advanced lactation knowledge and skills, and is labor-intensive and time-consuming (Meier et al., 2010).

In our combined human milk (HM) clinical-research program at Rush University Medical Center, we have used NICU-based breast-feeding peer counselors (BPCs), mothers of former very preterm infants who provided milk for their hospitalized infants, to provide evidence-based, NICU-specific lactation care (Meier, Engstrom, & Rossman, 2013; Meier, Patel, Bigger, Rossman, & Engstrom, 2012; Rossman, Greene, Kratovil, & Meier, 2012). The relationship between the new mother and the BPC begins in the early post-birth period as the BPCs share their stories of having a very preterm infant in the NICU, why they decided to provide milk, any complications their infant had, and show pictures of their infant in the NICU and as a growing and thriving child. As mothers of hospitalized NICU infants typically do not have the benefit of learning from someone who has been in a similar situation, new mothers find it therapeutic to talk with someone who has firsthand knowledge of how difficult it can be to cope with the emotional stress of having had a traumatic birth, as well as provide milk for and cope with the emotional stress of having an infant hospitalized in the NICU (Rossman et al., 2013; Rossman, Greene, & Meier, 2014).

Mothers receive several benefits from working with NICU-based BPCs. Our several studies about the BPC role indicate that it is highly valued by NICU families and NICU health care providers, and mothers indicate that the shared experience of having an infant in the NICU, rather than any demographic similarities, is at the heart of the BPC-new mother relationship (Rossman et al., 2011; Rossman, Engstrom, & Meier, 2012; Rossman et al., 2013; Rossman et al., 2014). Mothers also rate the peer and emotional support they receive from their day-to-day interactions with the BPCs as the most positive aspect of being in the NICU (Rossman et al., 2014). Mothers appreciate the lactation information, assistance, and support the BPCs gave them. The BPCs also provide therapeutic emotional support in the form of chatting, an informal communication that demonstrates to the new mothers that the BPCs care for and about them. Mothers feel that the insights they gain from these discussions with the BPCs help them establish, maintain, and enhance their confidence as a mother. Mothers are also encouraged by the BPCs in their efforts to develop a relationship with their infants by focusing on strategies (infant care-giving, skin-to-skin holding, providing milk) to become advocates for their infants. Through these interactions, mothers develop a resilience that indicate that they have begun adapting to NICU stressors, display inner strength in coping with the adversities of the preterm birth and NICU hospitalization, and are beginning to develop a maternal identity. By acting as role models, the BPCs also help mothers address future problems related to their infant's discharge from the NICU and give mothers hope that their lives will settle into a new normal as a family (Rossman et al., 2014).

Mothers also have faith in the healing properties of their milk for their preterm infants (Rossman et al., 2013). Mothers have faith that their milk is not just "good" for their infants; rather, they equate providing milk with "giving life" to their infants, mitigating the effects of complications, keeping their infants healthy and stable, and with helping themselves begin the processes of healing and addressing the feelings of failure and guilt associated with the premature birth.

Mothers' "faith in the milk" to achieve these outcomes is a maternal motivator to continue providing milk, even for those mothers who had not intended to provide milk initially, or who experience the paradox of disliking pumping, but wanting to provide their milk. Mothers hear the information about providing milk and pumping, they find hope listening to the BPCs' stories, which enable them to see the "possibilities" of their situations, and act with faith that their milk will do what they were told it would do. The mothers' faith in their milk is rewarded when they witness the positive impact their milk has on their infant's health, which in turn strengthens their faith and becomes a powerful motivator to continue pumping.

Peer support and role modeling by the BPCs, has been important for new mothers in our NICU, to help them provide for and become advocates for their infants, to help them become a mother to their infants, to give them hope about the possibilities of a normal life with their children, and to develop the inner strength and resilience necessary to cope with their infants' hospitalization.

References

Callen, J., & Pinelli, J. (2005). A review of the literature examining the benefits and challenges, incidence and duration, and barriers to breastfeeding in preterm infants. *Advances in Neonatal Care, 5*(2), 72-88. doi:10.1016/j.adnc.2004.12.003

Cregan, M. D., De Mello, T. R., Kershaw, D., McDougall, K., & Hartmann, P. E. (2002). Initiation of lactation in women after preterm delivery. *Acta Obstetrica Gynecolica Scandinavia, 81*(9), 870-877. doi: 10.1034/j.1600-0412.2002.810913.x

Hill, P. D., Aldag, J. C., Chatterton, R. T., & Zinaman, M. (2005a). Comparison of milk output between mothers of preterm and term infants: The first 6 weeks after birth. *Journal of Human Lactation, 21*(1), 22-30. doi: 10.1177/0890334404272407

Hill, P. D., Aldag, J. C., Chatterton, R. T., & Zinaman, M. (2005b). Primary and secondary mediators' influence on milk output in lactating mothers of preterm and term infants. *Journal of Human Lactation, 21*(2), 138-150. doi: 10.1177/0890334405275403

Lessen, R., & Crivelli-Kovach, A. (2007). Prediction of initiation and duration of breast-feeding for neonates admitted to the neonatal intensive care unit. *Journal of Perinatal and Neonatal Nursing, 21*(3), 256-266. doi: 10.1097/01.JPN.0000285817.51645.73

Meier, P. P., Engstrom, J. L., Patel, A. L., Jegier, B. L., & Bruns, N. E. (2010). Improving the use of human milk during and after the NICU stay. *Clinics in Perinatology, 37*(1), 217–245. doi:10.1016/j.clp.2010.01.013

Meier, P. P., Engstrom, J. L., & Rossman, B. (2013). Breastfeeding peer counselors as direct lactation care providers in the Neonatal Intensive Care Unit. *Journal of Human Lactation, 29*(3), 313-322. doi:10.1177/0890334413482184

Meier, P. P., Patel, A. L., Bigger, H. R., Rossman, B., & Engstrom, J. L. (2012). Supporting breastfeeding in the Neonatal Intensive Care Unit: Rush Mother's Milk Club as a case study of evidence-based care. *Pediatric Clinics of North America*, 60, 209-226. doi:10.1016/j.pcl.2012.10.007

Rossman, B., Engstrom, J. L., Meier, P. P., Vonderheid, S. C., Norr, K. F., & Hill, P. D. (2011). "They've walked in my shoes:" Mothers of very low birth weight infants and their experiences with breastfeeding peer counselors in the neonatal intensive care unit. *Journal of Human Lactation, 27*(1), 14-24. doi: 10.1177/0890334410390046

Rossman, B., Engstrom, J. L., & Meier, P. P. (2012). Healthcare providers' perceptions of breastfeeding peer counselors in the Neonatal Intensive Care Unit. *Research in Nursing and Health, 35*(5), 460-474. doi: 10.1002/nur.21496.

Rossman, B., Greene, M. M., Kratovil, A., & Meier, P. P. (2012). Supporting mothers of infants in the NICU. In V. Thorley & M. C. Vickers (Eds.), *The 10th step and beyond: Mother support for breastfeeding*. Amarillo, TX: Hale Publishing.

Rossman, B., Kratovil, A. L., Greene, M. M., Engstrom, J. L., & Meier, P. P. (2013). "I have faith in my milk:" The meaning of milk for mothers of very low birth weight infants hospitalized in the neonatal intensive care unit. *Journal of Human Lactation, 29*(3), 359-365. doi:10.1177/0890334413484552

Rossman, B., Greene, M. M., & Meier, P. P. (2014). The role of peer support in the development of maternal identity for "NICU moms". (Manuscript under review)

"One Nipple at a Time": IBCLCs' Strategies for Success and Recommendations for Improving Interprofessional Collaboration

Erica H. Anstey

Research suggests that a fragmented health care system has a negative impact on the provision of optimal support for breastfeeding dyads (Arthur, Saenz, & Replogle, 2003; Krogstrand & Parr, 2005; Register, Eren, Lowdermilk, Hammond, & Tully, 2000; Schanler, Schultz, & Wyble, 1999; Sleutel, Schultz, & Wyble, 2007; Szucs, Miracle, Rosenman, 2009; Taveras et al., 2004). The AAP recommends that the newborn be evaluated within 48 to 72 hours of hospital discharge by a qualified health care professional to assess breastfeeding. However, only 27% of maternity care facilities in the U.S. "provide hospital discharge care including a phone call to the patient's home, opportunity for follow-up visit, and referral to community breastfeeding support" (Centers for Disease Control and Prevention, 2011). Mothers often struggle to obtain breastfeeding support upon discharge from the hospital (U.S. Department of Health and Human Services, 2011).

While pediatricians, nurses, and other medical professionals sometimes help with breastfeeding issues, lactation consulting is growing as a profession to meet the breastfeeding support needs of mothers.

International Board Certified Lactation Consultants (IBCLCs) are internationally recognized health care professionals specifically trained to manage breastfeeding and human lactation (International Lactation Consultant Association, 2011). Studies have found that women who deliver their babies in hospitals that provide lactation support from an IBCLC have higher rates of any, and exclusive, breastfeeding compared to hospitals that do not have IBCLC lactation professionals (Bonuck, Trombley, Freeman, & McKee, 2005; Castrucci, Hoover, Lim, & Maus, 2006; Rishel & Sweeney, 2005). The role of the lactation consultant within the health care system has the potential to bridge disciplines and improve breastfeeding success rates. However, lactation consultants' perspectives on professional breastfeeding support roles within an interprofessional context have not been explored.

In this dissertation study, I was interested in understanding the perspective of lactation consultants who work with breastfeeding families and the barriers they face as professionals. The purpose of this presentation was to discuss the results related to IBCLCs' perspectives on role and strategies for negotiating barriers in their profession and their recommendations for improving coordination of care to optimize breastfeeding support.

Method

Following a grounded-theory methodological approach, I recruited participants using purposive and snowball sampling methods. Participants were eligible if they were currently credentialed IBCLCs practicing in Florida, age 18 or older, English-speaking, and not practicing only in a neonatal intensive care unit (NICU) setting. IBCLCs who work only with infants in the NICU face distinct issues that differ from those who work with normal, healthy newborns.

Most interviews took place in person (n=23) while some were conducted over the phone (n=5) or via Skype (n=2). Interviews lasted between 70 minutes and 2 ½ hours with an average of about 2 hours. Data were digitally recorded, professionally transcribed, and coded and analyzed in Atlas.ti to identify emergent themes. I kept careful notes about the coding process and the development of themes to determine when theoretical saturation was reached by applying the constant-comparative method during axial coding. After 28 interviews, saturation was reached. However, two additional interviews were conducted to confirm saturation; no new codes were added. I applied symbolic interactionism as a guiding theoretical framework to examine issues related to role and identity.

Findings

I interviewed 30 currently certified, female IBCLCs who practice in a range of settings that include hospitals, private practices, pediatric offices, breastfeeding centers, and WIC clinics. Participants ranged in age from 34 to 70 (M=52) and self-identified as white (n=22), Hispanic (n=7), and Asian (n=1). Half of the participants (n=15) were allied health professionals whose backgrounds included the IBCLC credential only, or included experience as peer counselors, or training in other health specialties. Of the remaining sample, 12 participants were nurses, and three were pediatricians.

Role Perception

IBCLCs perceived their role as multifaceted, represented by six emergent themes: educator, breastfeeding expert, health care team member, emotional support, holistic approach, and empowering mothers. Participants described their professional approach to working with mothers and babies as more holistic compared to other providers. One participant described the role of the IBCLC as the missing link between pediatricians and obstetricians, "because they can be very focused, and I think we are very global." One participant summed up the multiple roles of the IBCLC:

> The role of the IBCLC is to empower women to have the choice to breastfeed, and to meet their breastfeeding goals, and to work with the rest of the community in which the woman lives, and other health professionals in making that choice possible. (WIC)

I also asked about the role of other providers in breastfeeding support. Despite being somewhat critical of physicians who are not current with evidence-based breastfeeding information and practices, the IBCLCs were also understanding of the limitations facing physicians, such as appointment times and other competing demands. While they believe that the role of other providers should include educating and supporting breastfeeding mothers, they also described the need for providers to refer to IBCLCs as the experts in breastfeeding management. One private practice IBCLC stated,

> I think that their number one role should be to refer out when there's a problem, unless they have extra training [. . .] I mean a family practice doctor wouldn't be doing a cardiac ultrasound on a patient that had a heart problem because that's not their area of expertise.

Role Impact

The theme of this conference is Forging Partnerships. The IBCLCs in this study shared insight into the barriers they face in forging partnerships with health care providers, as well as ideas for improving collaboration. Participants frequently expressed their frustration with other providers who don't refer mothers to IBCLCs early enough. When these mothers finally access a lactation consultant, they feel that the care results in what one participant called "damage control." IBCLCs also grappled with feeling that they are not respected by other health care professionals, and are not acknowledged as the experts in lactation management. One IBCLC commented,

> Well, I'm second guessed. I am not really seen in the medical community. I think they still view us as lay-people [. . .] I mean, we're board certified, but that doesn't mean anything. You don't really have the flexibility to just pick up the phone and say, "Hey Doc, I need to have a consult with you." You just don't have that. It's not available to you. (Private Practice)

In contrast, when IBCLCs felt respected, many of the barriers they typically encountered in managing breastfeeding problems were eliminated, and subsequently, they believed that mothers had easier access to support.

Strategies for Successful Partnerships

Participants described various communication tactics with other providers as essential to building rapport, educating about breast-feeding, and cultivating collaborative relationships. Communication strategies, such as sharing evidence-based articles and sending reports to mother's physicians, reflect IBCLCs' perceived role as educators. While many described this communication with other providers as typically one-sided, some participants felt that open communication eventually led to positive relationships with physicians and nurses who were open to learning from them and respected their expertise.

Other recommendations for improving interprofessional collaboration included standardized breastfeeding education, interdisciplinary networking opportunities, institutional policies that value breast-feeding, and a focus on developing relationships to improve service utilization and referral processes. Participants often emphasized the need for a team-based approach and better overall coordination. This quote reflects this common perspective:

> Understanding that we're all overlapping, and that we all need to be respected [. . .] I don't know how to fix a lot of things [. . .] I need my team. But I do know that when I say, "You need to look into this because this is what I think it might be," that that should be taken seriously. As seriously as if the pediatrician calls me and says, "This baby is not transferring. I need you to do a really good assessment." Not that I would ever do anything less, but that my word should matter as much as theirs. Understanding that I have different roles, and that I'm limited in what I can do, as they are [. . .] We are their allies. We're not their enemies. (Private Practice)

Participants believe that collaboration will improve outcomes, and lead to more effective and efficient delivery of breastfeeding support services.

Discussion

IBCLCs come from a range of backgrounds and work in a variety of settings, and thus, experience different barriers. However, as the lactation management experts, IBCLCs have a unique role to play on the maternal-infant health care team. Better integration into the health care team, and improved interprofessional collaboration, may better enable the IBCLC to successfully manage lactation problems and support breastfeeding mothers. One IBCLC described her dedication to overcoming barriers in this way:

> Why do I keep banging my head against the wall? Because one nipple at a time, we're going to make a difference for lifelong health to not just babies, but mommies [. . .] I probably come from an evidence-based core philosophy. I come from an empowerment core

philosophy. I come from a team-approach core philosophy. And we will someday be there. (WIC)

In conclusion, IBCLCs offer a unique perspective on interprofessional collaborative approaches to breastfeeding support which should be included in future programs and interventions aimed at quality improvement in the care of breastfeeding mothers and infants.

References

Arthur, C. R., Saenz, R., & Replogle, W. H. (2003). Breastfeeding education, treatment, and referrals by female physicians. *Journal of Human Lactation, 19*(3), 303-309.

Bonuck, K. A., Trombley, M., Freeman, K., & McKee, D. (2005). Randomized, controlled trial of a prenatal and postnatal lactation consultant intervention on duration and intensity of breastfeeding up to 12 months. *Pediatrics, 116*(6), 1413-1426.

Castrucci, B. C., Hoover, K. L., Lim, S., & Maus, K. C. (2006). A comparison of breastfeeding rates in an urban birth cohort among women delivering infants at hospitals that employ and do not employ lactation consultants. *Journal of Public Health Management and Practice, 12*(6), 578-585.

Centers for Disease Control and Prevention. (2011). mPINC Results. Retrieved July 16, 2015, from http://www.cdc.gov/breastfeeding/data/mpinc/results-tables.htm

International Lactation Consultant Association. (2011). Position paper on the role and impact of the IBCLC. Retrieved July 16, 2015, from http://www.ilca.org/files/resources/ilca_publications/Role%20%20Impact%20of%20the%20IBCLC-webFINAL_08-15-11.pdf

Krogstrand, K. S., & Parr, K. (2005). Physicians ask for more problem-solving information to promote and support breastfeeding. *Journal of the American Dietetic Association, 105*(12), 1943-1947.

Register, N., Eren, M., Lowdermilk, D., Hammond, R., & Tully, M. R. (2000). Knowledge and attitudes of pediatric office nursing staff about breastfeeding. *Journal of Human Lactation, 16*(3), 210-215.

Rishel, P. E., & Sweeney, P. (2005). Comparison of breastfeeding rates among women delivering infants in military treatment facilities with and without lactation consultants. *Military Medicine, 170*(5), 435-438.

Schanler, R. J., O'Connor, K. G., & Lawrence, R. A. (1999). Pediatricians' practices and attitudes regarding breastfeeding promotion. *Pediatrics, 103*(3), E35.

Sleutel, M., Schultz, S., & Wyble, K. (2007). Nurses' views of factors that help and hinder their intrapartum care. *Journal of Obstetric, Gynecologic, & Neonatal Nursing, 36*(3), 203-211.

Szucs, K. A., Miracle, D. J., & Rosenman, M. B. (2009). Breastfeeding knowledge, attitudes, and practices among providers in a medical home. *Breastfeeding Medicine, 4*(1), 31-42.

Taveras, E. M., Li, R., Grummer-Strawn, L., Richardson, M., Marshall, R., Rego, V. H., . . . Lieu, T. A. (2004). Mothers' and clinicians' perspectives on breastfeeding counseling during routine preventive visits. *Pediatrics, 113*(5), e405-e411.

U.S. Department of Health and Human Services. (2011). *The Surgeon General's Call to Action to Support Breastfeeding.* Washington, DC: U.S. Department of Health and Human Services, Office of the Surgeon General.

Differentiating the Research on Peer/Lactation Counselors and IBCLC's: Focus on International Board Certified Lactation Consultants (IBCLCs)

Ellen Chetwynd and Catherine Sullivan

Breastfeeding support for women and children in the United States is going through a pivotal transition period. Under the Women's Preventative Services Guidelines, the Affordable Care Act specifically mandates that insurance providers cover the cost of "Comprehensive lactation support and counseling by a trained provider during pregnancy and/or in the postpartum period" (Rangel, 2009). With this legislation, the federal government has recognized the importance of breastfeeding as a health care intervention, and acknowledged that women need support from trained providers when breastfeeding problems develop. However, the definition of "trained provider" is broad, and gives little guidance to insurers on who to recognize as trained providers of medical lactation counseling.

There are three broad types of lactation support: peer counselors, primary health care providers, and lactation-specific management. For the sake of clarity, this presentation will focus on International Board Certified Lactation Consultants (IBCLC) as the credentialed providers of medical lactation consulting. There are distinct differences in scope and training between IBCLCs and peer counselors.

Most importantly, peer counselors need to have breastfed in order to provide peer support. They are expected to access and utilize their own experience with breastfeeding in order to help others. IBCLCs are trained health care professionals and as such, utilize the extensive education they received in human lactation and management of breastfeeding difficulties to help breastfeeding women with problems. The scope of a peer counselor is limited to encouragement and minor problem solving, while an IBCLC is the referral point for medical lactation counseling.

The care provided by an IBCLC is also different from that given by a primary care provider (PCP). An IBCLC must practice in a clinical setting, under the supervision of an experienced IBCLC for 300 to1000 hours, as well as completing 90 hours of education specifically on human lactation and medical lactation consulting before sitting for an internationally administered exam. While the PCP coordinates and supervises the care of the breastfeeding mother and baby, they often do not have the training to address the more complex breastfeeding difficulties. Additionally, a visit with a PCP will typically last 20 to 40 minutes, and includes a wide range of health care topics, while an IBCLC will take 60 to 90 minutes in an outpatient visit to work specifically on breastfeeding. While many PCPs recognize the expertise of the IBCLC, and will refer their breastfeeding patients for support, insurance providers inconsistently recognize and reimburse families for the care they receive from IBCLCs (Chetwynd, Meyer, Stuebe, Costello, & Labbok, 2013).

Advocating for breastfeeding support by IBCLCs requires an understanding of the evidence base. This presentation will summarize current research on IBCLCs, as well as the outcomes from IBCLC interventions to provide clarity as the breastfeeding community moves toward consensus on the definition of lactation support. Readers should refer Catherine Sullivan's presentation, "Differentiating the Research on Peer/Lactation Counselors and IBCLC's: Focus on Peer/Lactation Counseling" for a discussion of peer support.

We found 23 reviews and meta-analyses that address professional breastfeeding support. However, none differentiated between types of professional providers. For instance, Britton et al. (Britton, McCormick, Renfrew, Wade, & King, 2007) reviewed 18 studies categorized as providing "professional support" interventions in a comparative Cochrane review of professional vs. peer support. Of the 18 interventions, two (11%) utilized IBCLCs. Hannula et al. (Hannula, Kaunonen, & Tarkka, 2008) specifically reviewed only professional support interventions. Their systemic review defined professional support as including IBCLCs, midwives, health visitors, nurses, or researchers. Six of their 31 studies included an intervention utilizing IBCLCs. As a final example, many health care advocates turn to the systemic evidence review and meta-analysis by the U.S. Preventative Services Task Force as a source of information about breastfeeding support (Guise et al., 2003). They looked specifically at primary-care-based interventions, and separated types of providers from their initial review of the literature for study inclusion. They categorized studies as being delivered by nurses, IBCLCs, physicians, or peer counselors. However, for the meta-analysis, they combined all these types of support together, and assessed type of care provided, rather than provider of care. If we look at the category of support most similar to actual IBCLC clinical support (phone or in-person support), there were seven studies in this category, and 29% of the interventions were delivered by IBCLCs. Clearly, the reviews and meta-analyses in the literature to date do not allow us to quantify the benefits of IBCLC-specific interventions.

In order to address this research gap, we searched the literature for articles on professional-breastfeeding-support interventions published since 2000. In order to most closely reflect the work of an IBCLC, we chose to exclude study interventions that did not allow for direct face-to-face postpartum contact, given our underlying assumption that IBCLCs do their best work when they are working face-to-face with a breastfeeding mother and baby. This meant that we excluded studies in which the intervention included only prenatal education, only telephone support postpartum, or situations in which the IBCLC was in the clinic, but not the provider of breastfeeding support. We included any intervention that: 1) identified IBCLC-specific care, 2) provided face-to-face care in the postpartum period, and 3) had at least three months of follow-up on breastfeeding duration, exclusivity, or both. The postpartum contact could be a problem-based consult or a standardized visit, it could occur in the hospital or the community setting, and it could be completed independently, or as a member of a team. While there had to be at least one contact that was face-to-face, this could be combined with telephone support. Finally, the IBCLCs could be a part of the health care system in which the intervention was taking place, or a research IBCLC who only worked with study participants as a member of the research team.

We found 10 studies that met our study criteria between 2000 and 2014 (Chertok, Shoham-Vardi, & Hallack, 2004; Gill, Reifsnider, & Lucke, 2007; Kools, Thijs, Kester, Van Den Brandt, & De Vries, 2005; Bonuck et al., 2014; Bonuck, Trombley, Freeman, & McKee, 2005; Pinelli, Atkinson, & Saigal, 2001; Su et al., 2007; Vari, Camburn, & Henly, 2000; Wambach et al., 2011; Witt, Smith, Mason, & Flocke, 2011). Six of the studies were randomized, controlled trials, one was a randomized trial, two were cohort designs, and one was quasi-experimental. Six used IBCLCs alone, and four used IBCLCs as a part of a team. Team members differed in each of the studies, including physicians, peer counselors, and medical and nursing students. Seven of the studies had visits that occurred in the hospital, as well as contact outside of the hospital, whether that was in person or on the phone. Five of the studies included prenatal contact, as well as postpartum contact. Only three interventions integrated the IBCLC into the health care setting, and the remainder utilized IBCLCs who were involved with the study participant from the perspective of an outside research provider.

Duration was measured in all 10 studies. Retrospective recall was utilized to determine the length of breastfeeding. The interim between contacts to determine duration varied between weekly, to as long as

3 months. Nine out of the 10 studies found a statistically significant improvement in duration with use of an IBCLC intervention.

Eight out of the 10 studies assessed exclusivity. All of them used self-report of infant intake to evaluate exclusivity. One study additionally measured intake at the breast during the follow-up study visits to verify reported intake. Six out of the eight studied reported a statistically significant improvement in exclusivity.

There were several study components that appeared to make a difference in the effectiveness of the intervention. The studies that incorporated an IBCLC into the health care system found more improvement than the interventions in which the IBCLCs came into the health care setting as research personnel. The study in which the IBCLC was dependent on a referral from a provider before she could provide care found no significant difference in exclusivity or duration. Finally, the study designs that incorporated a standardized IBCLC visit within the first two weeks, but allowed for continued support from the IBCLC as needed were among the most successful interventions.

In conclusion, IBCLC interventions are effective in prolonging exclusive breastfeeding and breastfeeding duration. However, the literature would benefit from more well-designed studies. Particular attention needs to be taken to insure that the interventions studied are financially feasible within our current health care setting. Finally, we need the research that will explore partnerships between IBCLCs and peer counselors. Breastfeeding women benefit from all types of breastfeeding support, but because there is the risk of lactation failure if appropriate care is not provided in a timely manner, the transition between peer support and more advanced lactation management needs to be as seamless as possible in order to maximize the benefits of both types of providers while providing the best support possible.

References

Bonuck, K., Stuebe, A., Barnett, J., Labbok, M. H., Fletcher, J., & Bernstein, P. S. (2014). Effect of primary care intervention on breastfeeding duration and intensity. *American Journal of Public Health, 104 Suppl 1*, S119-S127. doi:10.2105/AJPH.2013.301360 [doi]

Bonuck, K. A., Trombley, M., Freeman, K., & McKee, D. (2005). Randomized, controlled trial of a prenatal and postnatal lactation consultant intervention on duration and intensity of breastfeeding up to 12 months. *Pediatrics, 116*(6), 1413-1426. doi:10.1542/peds.2005-0435

Britton, C., McCormick, F. M., Renfrew, M. J., Wade, A., & King, S. E. (2007). Support for breastfeeding mothers. *Cochrane Database of Systematic Reviews (Online), (1)*(1), CD001141. doi:10.1002/14651858. CD001141.pub3

Chertok, I. R., Shoham-Vardi, I., & Hallack, M. (2004). Four-month breastfeeding duration in postcesarean women of different cultures in the israeli negev. *Journal of Perinatal & Neonatal Nursing, 18*(2), 145-160.

Chetwynd, E., Meyer, A. M., Stuebe, A., Costello, R., & Labbok, M. (2013). Recognition of international board certified lactation consultants by health insurance providers in the united states: Results of a national survey of lactation consultants. *Journal of Human Lactation: Official Journal of International Lactation Consultant Association, 29*(4), 517-526. doi:10.1177/0890334413499974; 10.1177/0890334413499974

Gill, S. L., Reifsnider, E., & Lucke, J. F. (2007). Effects of support on the initiation and duration of breastfeeding. *Western Journal of Nursing Research, 29*(6), 708-723. doi:10.1177/0193945906297376

Guise, J. M., Palda, V., Westhoff, C., Chan, B. K., Helfand, M., Lieu, T. A., & U.S. Preventive Services Task Force. (2003). The effectiveness of primary care-based interventions to promote breastfeeding: Systematic evidence review and meta-analysis for the US preventive services task force. *Annals of Family Medicine, 1*(2), 70-78.

Hannula, L., Kaunonen, M., & Tarkka, M. T. (2008). A systematic review of professional support interventions for breastfeeding. *Journal of Clinical Nursing, 17*(9), 1132-1143. doi:10.1111/j.1365-2702.2007.02239.x

Kools, E. J., Thijs, C., Kester, A. D., Van Den Brandt, P. A., & De Vries, H. (2005). A breastfeeding promotion and support program a randomized trial in the netherlands. *Preventive Medicine, 40*(1), 60-70. doi:10.1016/j.ypmed.2004.05.013

Pinelli, J., Atkinson, S. A., & Saigal, S. (2001). Randomized trial of breastfeeding support in very low-birth-weight infants. *Archives of Pediatrics & Adolescent Medicine, 155*(5), 548-553.

Rangel, C. (2009). Health care bill-H.R. 3590: Patient Protection and Affordable Care Act, 2010. Retrieved from http://housedocs,house. gov/energycommerce/ppacacon.pdf

Su, L. L., Chong, Y. S., Chan, Y. H., Chan, Y. S., Fok, D., Tun, K. T., . . . Rauff, M. (2007). Antenatal education and postnatal support strategies for improving rates of exclusive breast feeding: Randomised controlled trial. *BMJ (Clinical Research Ed.), 335*(7620), 596. doi:10.1136/bmj.39279.656343.55

Vari, P. M., Camburn, J., & Henly, S. J. (2000). Professionally mediated peer support and early breastfeeding success. *The Journal of Perinatal Education: An ASPO/Lamaze Publication, 9*(1), 22-30. doi:10.1624/105812400X87473

Wambach, K. A., Aaronson, L., Breedlove, G., Domian, E. W., Rojjanasrirat, W., & Yeh, H. W. (2011). A randomized controlled trial of breastfeeding support and education for adolescent mothers. *Western Journal of Nursing Research, 33*(4), 486-505. doi:10.1177/0193945910380408

Witt, A. M., Smith, S., Mason, M. J., & Flocke, S. A. (2011). Integrating routine lactation consultant support into a pediatric practice. *Breastfeeding Medicine: The Official Journal of the Academy of Breastfeeding Medicine.* doi:10.1089/bfm.2011.0003

CHAPTER 26

Breastfeeding and Health Care Personnel: The SLP's Role in Breastfeeding

Amber Valentine

The Speech-Language Pathologist is often seen in settings as the "go-to" for infants with feeding difficulties, predominantly for bottle-feeding or feeding aversions. In today's society, with breast-feeding becoming more and more "the norm," the SLP has become more involved in the area of feeding assessment with not only bottle-fed infants, but infants who are attempting breastfeeding as well. The SLP brings an interesting background to the area of breastfeeding with knowledge of the oral mechanism, infant respiratory system, and swallowing mechanisms. In many NICU and pediatric facilities, the SLP is now providing pre-feeding readiness assessments on infants, and by doing these, allowing many infants to get in on the ground floor with breastfeeding. These infants in the NICU and early pediatric setting can be provided with more opportunities to become successful breastfeeders, especially those infants who were previously thought to be unable to complete this task. As the literature shows, it is critical to provide human milk as soon as possible to these fragile infants in NICU. By allowing them to have earlier opportunities at the breast, they will be more likely to become not only successful breastfeeders, but more successful feeders for a lifetime.

In this presentation, we discuss how the SLP can provide more opportunities for these infants. With pre-feeding readiness assessments, along with early intervention, we can work along with NICU nursing staff, neonatologists, and lactation counselors to provide these infants with the best chance to succeed. The SLP can work with infants with feeding difficult to differentiate positioning needs, supplementation needs when necessary, oral stimulation when needed to be provided, suck training for infants, and compensatory techniques to help the infant and mother pace when possible to provide with more opportunities.

In many facilities, it is becoming more and more difficult for the lactation specialist to cover all areas of infants attempting to breastfeed. By working in conjunction with other disciplines, we can raise our breast-feeding success, not just in our own town, state, or at the national level, but can help spread breastfeeding success worldwide. At Baptist Health Lexington, our current NICU population has had more infants with other significant difficulties (cleft, syndromes, etc.) be discharged breastfeeding more successfully than bottle- feeding.

Forging Partnerships to Increase Community Support for Women, Children, and Families

Breastfeeding is a socially and culturally based behavior. Women generally need the help of others to succeed with breastfeeding. This section explores several parts of our environment that deserve attention as potential partners.

Section IVa

Breastfeeding in the Community: Sharing Health

The Breastfeeding Conversation: Forging Partnerships through Hermeneutic Dialogue

Jane Grassley

B reastfeeding advocacy involves forging synergistic partnerships with individuals and groups who represent diverse interests. Their understanding of, and priorities related to, breastfeeding support may be quite different than mine. For example, as a nurse of several decades, I value breastfeeding not only for its health benefits, but as an embodied relationship between a mother and her child (Barclay et al., 2012). However, if I am advocating for breastfeeding support in a business setting, I need to understand that business values reducing waste, cutting costs, and increasing profit (Wright, 2013). So how do I begin to forge a partnership with business, whose priorities seem so different than mine? In this paper, I explore Gadamerian hermeneutics as a useful framework for developing these partnerships through the concepts of dialogue or hermeneutic conversation, horizon, history, and language.

H. G. Gadamer was a German philosopher whose life spanned the 20th century (1900-2002). Hermeneutics involves the interpretation of texts, which Gadamer broadened to include life experiences, such as a breastfeeding a child (1999/1960). The ability to understand or interpret a text (e.g., breastfeeding and breastfeeding advocacy) takes place through a dialogue guided by genuine questions and answers that invite a collaborative exploration of the text, rather than just seeking information (Phillips, 2007).

The purpose of hermeneutic dialogue is to understand the horizon or standpoint of our conversational partners. Gadamer defined horizon as "the range of vision that includes everything that can be seen from a particular point of view" (1999/1960, p. 302). Horizons are formed by an individual's personal, professional, and sociocultural history of, and language about, a particular text, such as breastfeeding. History, as a compilation of "past experiences, family, culture, and historical tradition, conditions the choices we make, and the problems we notice" (Grassley & Nelms, 2008, p. E57). We develop a language about the text from our history; our language in turn structures how we view our experiences (Gadamer, 1999/1960), forming the horizon that we bring to breastfeeding advocacy. As we take the time to engage in a hermeneutic dialogue in order to understand a potential partner's horizon, we begin to forge synergistic partnerships that can make a difference for women's health. Gadamer (1999/1960) called this process a "fusion of horizons" (p. 306).

The breastfeeding conversation provides a model for breastfeeding advocates who want to engage in meaningful dialogue with a variety of conversational partners: individual mothers and their families, mother-to-mother organizations, legislators and other political leaders, health care professionals, the media, and businesses (see Figure 1). Conversational partners bring their history and language to their individual interpretation of a text. As they dialogue about the text, a fusion of horizons may occur. Grassley and Nelms (2008) first defined the breastfeeding conversation as "a hermeneutic encounter that takes place in the early postpartum and encompasses a text (particular feeding), conversational partners (the mother, her newborn, and the nurse), and an interpretation of the text by the conversational partners as effective or ineffective breastfeeding" (p. E58). How a mother inter-prets a feeding affects her breastfeeding confidence. Conceptualizing breastfeeding support as a hermeneutic dialogue with a mother and her newborn revolutionized my work as a lactation consultant and nurse. For this paper, I examine the breastfeeding conversation as a guide to engaging employers in a dialogue about implementing business policies that support and protect breastfeeding.

Several assumptions guided this conceptualization of the breast-feeding conversation. First, as a text breastfeeding advocacy involves championing and upholding women's choices to breastfeed, particularly in the workplace and in public. Our focus is to transform the work environment so that women have an easier time fulfilling their breastfeeding goals (Roy & Oludaja, 2009). Second, all conversational partners are active participants in the dialogue and bring a context or horizon formed by their history and language to the breastfeeding conversation. We need to be aware, particularly, of their priorities and shape our language about breastfeeding in ways that engage them in the give and take of genuine dialogue. Third, in advocating for breast-feeding protection in the workplace, we must be open to listening to viewpoints about breastfeeding that may challenge our own (Roy & Oludaja, 2009). Finally, we can empower women to engage in dialogue with their employers.

As a first step in the breastfeeding conversation, I need to define the text (breastfeeding and employment). For this discussion, breast-feeding and employment, as text, includes why breastfeeding support is good for business, what women need to return to work and continue breastfeeding, and how employers can implement supportive work-place policies. At a minimum, these might include a break time every 3 hours, and a clean, private (non-bathroom) place to express milk. Some employers provide worksite lactation programs that include access to information, breast pumps, and lactation consultant services (Wright, 2013).

I also need to reflect upon the horizon that I bring to the conversation, and identify my preconceptions about employers, breastfeeding, and combining working and breastfeeding. Gadamer (1999/1960) argued that our prejudices, or ways of viewing the world, influence how we interpret a text. In order to understand a text, we need to first understand our own history with the text. For example, my history with breastfeeding and employment does not include personal experience, but is limited to offering professional support to working women. My language about breastfeeding reflects a personal and professional belief in breastfeeding as primarily relational and embodied, as well as providing lifelong health benefits. This is not the language of business. Business priorities include language about profit, productivity, increased employee retention, and decreased employee recidivism (Wright, 2013). As I prepare for engaging employers as conversational partners, I need to be able to address their priorities using their language as we dialogue about breastfeeding and employment.

Individual employers bring a history and language about breastfeeding and employment that influence their interpretation of breastfeeding support in the workplace. Women bring a history grounded in their family's experiences with breastfeeding, their previous experiences breastfeeding their children, and their birth experiences (Grassley & Nelms, 2008). Their history may include personal experiences with combining breastfeeding and employment, as a mother, or with past employees. Men also bring a history grounded in family breastfeeding experiences, either from their mothers or their current family. They have a history and language about the place of breastfeeding support in the work environment. The nature of these experiences, whether positive or negative, forms the horizon they bring to the conversation.

The language of current federal and state laws impacts the dialogue. The Patient Protection and Affordable Care Act, passed in 2010, states that employers with more than 50 employees must provide reasonable, unpaid break time, and a private, non-bathroom place for a woman to express human milk up to her child's first birthday. Twenty-four states, the **District of Columbia,** and **Puerto Rico** have laws related to breastfeeding in the workplace. Oregon's law is considered a model because women are allowed 30 minutes to express their human milk for every 4 hours worked (National Conference of State Legislatures, 2011).

We access our conversational partners' horizon by asking questions and listening for the language of their concerns. For example, if employee productivity is a priority, and they are concerned about time lost due to mothers expressing milk, I can provide them with information about how breastfeeding families have fewer unscheduled personal days or absences due to infant illness (Lactation Navigation, 2014). Employers may use the language of costs, which can be addressed through talking about the savings in health care costs, and through increased employee retention. Cigna (2000) found that their lactation support program saved a total of $240,000 annually in health care expenses for breastfeeding mothers and their children. The desired outcome of this dialogue is a fusion of horizons that results in the implementation of supportive workplace breastfeeding policies. We can also engage individual women in a dialogue about breastfeeding and employment in order to empower them as advocated for supportive workplace policies.

To create a better tomorrow for mothers and their families, breastfeeding advocates need to forge partnerships with a variety of conversational partners: individual mothers and their families, mother-to-mother groups, legislators and other political leaders, health care professionals, the media, and businesses. The breastfeeding conversation through its concepts of dialogue, history and language, and fusion of horizons offers a model for engaging in meaningful dialogue that can promote, support, and protect breastfeeding in a global context.

References

Barclay, L., Longman, J., Schmied, V., Sheehan, A., Rolfe, M., Burns, E., & Fenwikc, J. (2012). The professionalising (sic) of breast feeding: Where are we a decade on? *Midwifery, 28*, 281-290. doi: 10.1016/j.midw.2011.12.011 Cigna. (2000). UCLA study of Cigna corporate lactation program proves that helping working moms breastfeed is good business. Retrieved from http://newsroom.cigna.com/article_display.cfm?article_id=37

Gadamer, H. G. (1999). *Truth and method.* (2nd ed.) (J. Weinsheimer & D. G. Marshall, Trans.).New York: Continuum. (Original work published 1960)

Grassley, J. S., & Nelms, T. P. (2008). The breastfeeding conversation: A philosophical exploration of support. *Advances in Nursing Science, 31*(4), E55-E66.

Lactation Navigation. (2014). *Why support breastfeeding?* Retrieved from http://lactationnav.com/why_support_breastfeeding.shtml

National Conference of State Legislatures. (2011). *Breastfeeding laws.* Retrieved from http://www.ncsl.org/research/health/breastfeeding-state-laws.aspx

Phillips, B. (2007). Nursing care and understanding the experience of others: A Gadamerian perspective. *Nursing Inquiry, 14*(1), 89-94.

Roy, A., & Oludaja, B. (2009). Hans-Georg Gadamer's Praxis: Implications for connection and action in communication studies. *Communication, Culture & Critique, 2*, 255-273. doi: 10.1111/j.1753-9137.2009.01038.x

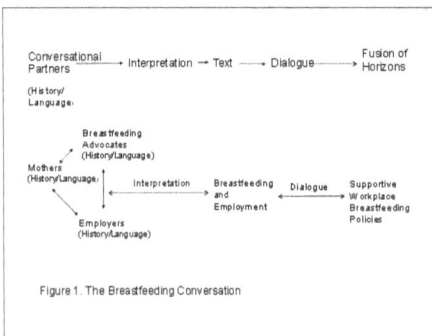

Figure 1. The Breastfeeding Conversation

Wright, W. (2013, November). *Returning to work without weaning.* Paper presented at Navigating the Bumps. iLactation online conference.

The Donor Human Milk Bank Registry: Exploring the Feasibility and Logistics of Development and Maintenance

Rachel M. Davis

Objectives

The purpose of this paper is to examine whether prenatal breast-feeding education, possibly mediated by breastfeeding self-efficacy, is associated with exclusive breastfeeding during the hospital stay. It will also address whether or not the impact of this association varies by race. Previous breastfeeding experience, hospital practices that support exclusive breastfeeding, and breastfeeding intention are observed as possible confounding factors.

Background

As rates of breastfeeding initiation are rising, the focus is increasing on methods to support improved duration. Research shows that prenatal breastfeeding promotion and education are helpful in terms of building confidence in new mothers, and preparing them for what to expect once their infant arrives. This paper is based on an ongoing evaluation of the Ready, Set, Baby (RSB) prenatal breastfeeding education program offered at the University of North Carolina Chapel Hill (UNC) Women's Hospital. Researchers are especially interested in program effectiveness and potential barriers to program participation as expansion of RSB is a future goal. Data collected during the 2013 summer phase was used to create this paper.

Method

The student researcher collaborated with the Carolina Global Breast-feeding Institute at UNC, and the UNC Women's Hospital, to conduct postpartum interviews with mothers who received prenatal care at UNC hospital, and who, therefore, were in the population that could have been offered the RSB educational sessions.

Results

Of the 76 women in the study, 28% identified as African American/ Non-Hispanic, 43% as Caucasian/Non-Hispanic, 1% as Asian/ Non-Hispanic, 3% as Other/Non-Hispanic, and 25% as Hispanic. About 61% of the population, the majority of whom were Caucasian, exclusively breastfed their infants during the entire hospital stay. Caucasian women also had the highest breastfeeding self-efficacy scores. The mean score among all women in the study was 60 out of 70; the score was slightly higher at 62.7 in women who exclusively breastfed. About 25% of women took a prenatal breastfeeding class to prepare for the arrival of their infant; 26% of whom exclusively breastfed. About 56% of all women reported having previously breastfed. Among this group, 60% exclusively breastfed their infants. The mean breastfeeding intention score was 7.9 out of 16. Yet the mean score for intention was lower (5.6) among exclusive breastfeeding women. African American and Hispanic women took prenatal breastfeeding classes more often than Caucasian women, had more previous breastfeeding experience, and higher intentions to breastfeed. All women in the study rated their exclusive breastfeeding supportive hospital care as "8 out of 10," or better. The mean score was 9.5 with Caucasian and Hispanic women reporting slightly higher ratings than African Americans.

Discussion and Conclusions

In contrast with most current research, this study did not strongly support the idea that factors of prenatal breastfeeding education, self-efficacy, previous breastfeeding experience, hospital practices that supported exclusive breastfeeding, and breastfeeding intention predict exclusive breastfeeding in the hospital. This study did not explain the racial/ethnic disparities that exist, and may need to be expanded to include a larger sample size to obtain significant findings. Other factors are important to consider, especially among minority populations and support, and breastfeeding education alone may not be enough for all women to achieve exclusive breastfeeding. The benefits of breastfeeding (and the costs of not breastfeeding) can be seen throughout the lifespan. By addressing racial/ethnic disparities among infants, researchers may also address racial/ethnic health disparities that exist in adults.

Poster Presentation Summary

The non-significant increased odds of EBF in the hospital with prenatal education found in this study add to the current body of literature that supports the idea that education and support are helpful in increasing EBF. Yet the racial/ethnic breakdown of prenatal education in this study, while not achieving significance, would seem to conflict with other studies because more African American and Hispanic women received education than Caucasian women, yet Caucasian women achieved higher rates of EBF than both minority populations.

Although some findings are supportive of current research, overall this study did not strongly support the idea that factors of prenatal breastfeeding education, breastfeeding self-efficacy, previous breastfeeding experience, EBF supportive hospital practices and breastfeeding intention contribute to EBF in the hospital. The higher rates of prenatal education class attendance and previous experience among Hispanic and African American women, the higher ratings of EBF supportive hospital care among Hispanic women, and higher intention scores among both minority populations (which all normally suggest higher rates of EBF), when compared to Caucasian women, concludes that other factors may need to be examined to address the racial/ethnic existing disparities. This study did not explain the racial/ethnic disparities that exist in achieving EBF, and this and future studies regarding factors contributing to EBF among racial/ethnic groups may need to be expanded to a larger sample size to obtain more significant findings.

Recommendations and Significance for Maternal and Child Health

Although the findings in this study did not strongly contribute to the literature on breastfeeding disparities, they did suggest that other factors are important to consider, and that support and prenatal breast-feeding education alone may not be enough for all women to achieve EBF. There were several factors in this study that have been proven to increase breastfeeding initiation and duration in a large number of other studies that did not do so here. When considering African American and Hispanic women, researchers have yet to determine why these women have lower breastfeeding rates. Outside factors that may, or may not, have been considered to date, such as deeper cultural implications, ideas, and norms that are preventing these women from achieving higher rates may need to be studied more in-depth. It is important to continue to conduct research in this area because there are factors that have yet to be determined that have the potential to affect whether or not a woman breastfeeds, and for how long. More importantly, the benefits of breastfeeding (and the costs of not breast-feeding) can be seen throughout the lifespan. By addressing racial/ethnic disparities in breastfeeding among infants, researchers may also address many of the racial/ethnic health disparities that exist in adults. The effects of this would not only be seen in health improvements among individuals, but may also positively impact an array of demographic (i.e., education level, income level, etc.), and economic factors (i.e., lower medical costs) in the U.S. society as a whole.

Forging New Partnerships for Milk Sharing: Preliminary Findings from the Anthropological Contexts of Milk Sharing (AnthroCOMS) Survey

Aunchalee Palmquist and Kirsten Doehler

Altruistic peer-to-peer milk sharing is an infant feeding practice that is growing in popularity in the U.S. (Akre, Gribble, & Minchin, 2011; Keim, McNamara, Dillon et al., 2014). Debates around the safety concerns of milk sharing have been well-documented in editorials, commentaries, and a growing body of research (Akre et al., 2011; Cassidy, 2012; Geraghty et al., 2013; Gribble, 2014c; Gribble & Hausman, 2012; Jones, 2013; Keim, McNamara, Jayadeva et al., 2014; Nelson, 2012; Rotstein, 2012). In an analysis of biomedical ethics *vis-à-vis* milk sharing, breastfeeding advocate Karleen Gribble notes that "health workers cannot ignore, dismiss, discount, or demonize peer sharing without acting unethically" (2012, p. 110). Health care providers are, thus, faced with the challenge of how to engage with the issue of milk sharing responsibly and ethically.

It is clear that health care providers and other types of breastfeeding supporters are ideally positioned to provide reliable information about the safety and risks involved in milk sharing. Yet, milk sharing involves more than simply weighing risks and benefits. What are some of the other needs and concerns of milk-sharing families? Can health care providers and other breastfeeding support personnel use their skills and expertise to address some of these needs?

The Anthropological Contexts of Milk Sharing Study (Anthro-COMS) is a mixed-method study designed to evaluate the biocultural context of milk sharing. This paper presents preliminary findings based on the survey data, which are related to understanding the broader social and emotional dimensions of milk sharing. The overall objective of this discussion session is to identify key areas for which new partnerships between milk sharing and those interested in breastfeeding support and advocacy might be forged.

Method

Following ethics approval by Elon University Institutional Review Board, an online survey was launched in September 2013. Respondents to the survey (N=1,116) were located in 15 countries with 76% donors and 24% recipients. The vast majority (94%) were based in the United States. The demographic profile of respondents was 99% female, 95% Caucasian, 94% married or in a domestic partnership, with an average age of 31, and an average of two children. Fifty-seven percent had some college, and 33% reported completing postgraduate studies. Employment status varied, with 34% employed full-time, 23% employed part-time, and 43% not employed at the time of the survey.

Respondents were included in the analyses if they were at least 18 years of age, had experience as a milk-sharing donor or recipient during their most recent lactation, were seeking milk for infant feeding, and were residing in the United States. Descriptive results and statistical analyses were conducted using SAS v. 93 software (SAS Institute, Cary, NC 2011). Two independent samples z-tests for proportions were executed to ascertain whether any differences between donor and recipient responses were statistically significant at p<0.05. We evaluated three domains, including multiple types of breastfeeding support, lactation assessment, and milk-sharing effect.

Results

The final subset of respondents (n=867) included 661 donors and 206 recipients from across the U.S. The average lifetime lactation for donors was 26 months, and the average for recipients was 20 months. There were no significant differences between donors' and recipients' median age, employment status, marital status, or number of pregnancies and births. Donors reported significantly higher levels of education and household income. The average age of the baby at most recent lactation was 5 months for donors, and 7 months for recipients. Recipients reported receiving milk from an average of 8 donors, and donors reported sharing milk with an average of three recipients. Donors reported expressing, on average, .33L of milk per day to share, and recipients reported feeding their babies on average .53L of milk per day. Donors reported sharing an estimated 40L of milk in total, while recipients reported feeding their babies, on average, 84L of shared donor milk.

Breastfeeding Support

Donors reported significantly greater breastfeeding support from spouses/partners, other family members, employers, and pediatricians. There were no statistically significant differences in reports of breastfeeding support for friends, other childcare providers, lactation consultants, doulas, midwives, nurses, and obstetrician/gynecologists. Online social networks were an important resource for breastfeeding support among 96% of respondents.

Lactation Assessment

The survey was used to collect information that might be typically used in a lactation assessment, including maternal medical history, and maternal and infant conditions associated with most recent lactation.

Donors reported significantly higher rates of mastitis, overactive milk ejection reflect, and plugged ducts. Recipients reported significantly higher rates of low milk supply, insufficient glandular tissue (IGT), taking medications contraindicated for breastfeeding, nipple or breast infection (other than mastitis), postpartum separation, cesarean birth, IVF/IUI, and postpartum depression associated with most recent lactation. Recipients also reported significantly higher rates of breast reduction surgery, history of depression, history of BMI >30, polycystic ovarian syndrome (PCOS), and hypothyroidism. There were no significant differences between donors and recipients reports of breastfeeding pain, Raynaud's Syndrome, vasospasm, or yeast infections. Recipients reported significantly higher rates of employing multiple complementary and alternative therapies for lactation, including herbal and prescription pharmaceutical galactagogues.

Milk Sharing Affect

Donors and recipients were asked to provide information about their feelings associated with milk sharing during their most recent lactation. Positive affect was measured as feeling "empowered," "happy," "confident," and "informed." Negative affect was measured as feeling "sad," "inadequate," "anxious," and "confused." Respondents were asked to indicate the frequency with which they experienced these feelings using a 5-point Likert Scale. Responses were dichotomized for analysis ("most of the time/always," and "half of the time/rarely/never"). There were no statistically significant differences between donors' and recipients' responses for feeling "informed." Donors reported significantly higher rates of feeling empowered, happy, and confident. Recipients reported significantly higher rates of feeling inadequate, sad, anxious, and confused.

Discussion

Milk sharing is a biocultural phenomenon that is inextricably linked with patterns of lactation and breastfeeding practices (Stuart-Macadam & Dettwyler, 1995). It also occurs in social contexts with particular cultural, historical, political economic, technological dimensions that shape the motivations, practices, meanings, and often the biology and well-being of those who are involved. In the United States, there are considerable structural barriers that make breastfeeding, as recommended by the World Health Organization (WHO, 2003), and the American Academy of Pediatrics (AAP, 2012), difficult, if not impossible. Common structural barriers in the U.S. include lack of paid maternity/parental leave, lack of employer accommodations for breastfeeding or expressing milk at work, lack of access to effective breastfeeding health care providers, hospital and birthing practices that are deleterious to breastfeeding, social stigma against public breastfeeding, and institutional racism.

In cases where parents are not able to breastfeed or provide breastmilk to their babies, human milk banks are one option for supporting exclusive breastmilk feedings. However, the Human Milk Banking Association of North America (HMBANA) milk banks currently have the capacity to only provide milk to the most medically fragile infants. Few hospitals cover the costs of banked donor milk, not all insurance companies cover the costs of banked donor milk, and the out-of-pocket cost of banked milk is prohibitively high for most families. Peer-to-peer milk sharing has expanded as a way to bridge the gap between the milk that HMBANA provides, and families who cannot access banked donor milk.

Improving breastfeeding outcomes is the obvious place to begin, in both reducing the demand for breastmilk within milk-sharing networks, and also increasing the potential donor pool to expand milk banking in the U.S. The data from our study also indicate that there are other important issues at play. Many of the patterns uncovered by our survey point to issues that warrant further investigation. Lower breastfeeding rates among recipients may be strongly associated with BMI >30, IGT, and perinatal mood disorders (Stuebe et al., 2014). Many recipients who are milk sharing are breastfeeding mothers who have tried to breastfeed, but have experienced low milk supply (Gribble, 2014a, 2014b; Perrin, Goodell, Allen, & Fogleman, 2014). These mothers are highly motivated to breastfeed, and value human milk for the many health benefits it provides (Gribble, 2014a). Not being able to breastfeed may exacerbate feelings of sadness, anxiety, and inadequacy, and these patterns are reflected in our data. Making mental health support an integral part of breastfeeding support is essential for these mothers, regardless of how they are supplementing their infants.

Greater negative feelings about milk sharing may also reflect a lack of health care provider support in coping with breastfeeding challenges, and making informed decisions about milk sharing. There are currently no guidelines available to assist families with navigating the risks of sharing milk outside of a milk bank, and most people who share milk do so without consulting a health care provider (Gribble, 2014). The stigma surrounding milk sharing, which is exacerbated by highly moralized risk messaging from various health authorities, may lead parents to avoid discussing questions about milk sharing with their health care providers, or disclosing that they are feeding their child with shared donor milk. Establishing guidelines for health care providers to follow, as well as opening pathways of communication so that health care providers may approach milk sharing through a lens of informed decision making, are essential to reducing the potential risks of milk sharing. Health care providers have an opportunity to advocate for universal access to banked donor milk for breastfed babies who require supplementation, and to promote donation to milk banks among mothers who may have a surplus of milk to give.

Milk sharing provides a number of opportunities for health care providers to contribute to better breastfeeding. The first step is finding ways to open respectful communication about the relative risks and benefits of all infant feeding alternatives so that parents are able to make informed decisions that are consistent with their child's health status and circumstances (Gribble & Hausman, 2012; WHO, 2003). More research is needed to better assess the risks of milk-sharing practices and the health outcomes of infants who receive donor milk, as well as the sociocultural context and lived experience of milk-sharing practices.

References

American Academy Academy (AAP). (2012). Breastfeeding and the Use of Human Milk. *Pediatrics, 129*(3), 2011–3552.

Akre, J. E., Gribble, K. D., & Minchin, M. (2011). Milk sharing: From private practice to public pursuit. *International Breastfeeding Journal, 6*(8), 1–3.

Cassidy, T. M. (2012). Making "milky matches": Globalization, maternal trust, and "lactivist" online networking. *Journal of the Motherhood Initiative, 3*(1), 226–240.

Geraghty, S. R., McNamara, K. A., Dillon, C. E., Hogan, J. S., Kwiek, J. J., & Keim, S. A. (2013). Buying human milk via the Internet: just a click away. *Breastfeeding Medicine, 8*(6), 474–478.

Gribble, K. D. (2014a). "A better alternative": Why women use peer-to-peer shared milk. *Breastfeeding Review, 22*(1), 11–21.

Gribble, K. D. (2014b). "I'm happy to be able to help:" Why women donate to a peer via Internet-based milk sharing networks. *Breastfeeding Medicine, 9*(5), 251–256.

Gribble, K. D. (2014c). Perception and management of risk in Internet-based peer-to-peer milk-sharing. *Early Child Development and Care, 184*(1), 84–98.

Gribble, K. D., & Hausman, B. L. (2012). Milk sharing and formula feeding: Infant feeding risks in comparative perspective? *The Australasian Medical Journal, 5*(5), 275–283.

Jones, F. (2013). Milk sharing: how it undermines breastfeeding. *Breastfeeding Review, 21*(3), 21–25.

Keim, S. A., McNamara, K. A., Dillon, C. E., Strafford, K., Ronau, R., McKenzie, L. B., & Geraghty, S. R. (2014). Breastmilk sharing: awareness and participation among women in the Moms2Moms Study. *Breastfeeding Medicine, 9*, 398–406.

Keim, S. A., McNamara, K. A., Jayadeva, C. M., Braun, A. C., Dillon, C. E., & Geraghty, S. R. (2014). Breast milk sharing via the Internet: The practice and health and safety considerations. *Maternal and Child Health Journal, 18*(6), 1471–1479.

Nelson, R. (2012). Breast milk sharing is making a comeback, but should it? *The American Journal of Nursing, 112*(6), 19–20.

Perrin, M. T., Goodell, L. S., Allen, J. C., & Fogleman, A. (2014). A mixed-methods observational study of human milk sharing communities on Facebook. *Breastfeeding Medicine, 9*(3), 128–134.

Rotstein, C. (2012). *Online social breast-working: Representations of breast milk sharing in the 21st Century*. University of Western Ontario - Electronic Thesis and Dissertation Repository. Retrieved from http://ir.lib.uwo.ca/etd/1029

Stuart-Macadam, P., & Dettwyler, K. A. (Eds.). (1995). *Breastfeeding: Biocultural perspectives*. New York: Aldine de Gruyter.

Stuebe, A. M., Horton, B. J., Chetwynd, E., Watkins, S., Grewen, K., & Meltzer-Brody, S. (2014). Prevalence and risk factors for early, undesired weaning attributed to lactation dysfunction. *Journal of Women's Health*, [e-pub ahead of print], doi: 10.1089/jwh.2013.4506.

WHO. (2003). *Global strategy for infant and young child feeding*. Geneva, Switzerland: World Health Organization. Retrieved from http://whqlibdoc.who.int/publications/2003/9241562218.pdf?ua=1

A V-formation Approach to Breastfeeding and Milk Sharing Families

Agustina Vidal

In the year 2000, I joined *"Project Mujeres* 2000," a microcredit program created and implemented by political science students for the benefit of women living in the Los Troncos slum of Buenos Aires. It wasn't long before I realized what a profound impact our presence was having on the community, for the simple fact that, for the first time in a long time, these women felt like they were being listened to. As social creatures, telling our stories is an act of affirmation, and when our stories move those around us to take positive steps, we feel real, relevant, and important. It is through this ripple effect that we transform ourselves, others, and our communities.

After two years of working in Los Troncos, I had learned a valuable lesson; namely, that social change, when not translated into social policy, is unstable and fragile. The women of Los Troncos had, in many ways, advanced their lives and the life of their community. However, their access to social and economic justice remained unchanged. This was because, despite their participation in *Mujeres*, there was still a lack of health, educational, and social policy.

Armed with this newfound knowledge, I migrated to the public sector, and from 2002 to 2006, held a position as a Congressional Aid, where I realized that public policies not birthed through collective storytelling are usually useless and harmful. Historically, the process toward social change has been an assembly line, much like Charlie Chaplin's *Modern Times*. Each actor works in his/her station, without knowledge of the final product.

This assembly-line model is often replicated throughout systems, and unfortunately, it has informed the model of care received by pregnant women, especially when it pertains to breastfeeding education and support. A woman typically learns about breastfeeding during a prenatal class; she later births in ways that impact or enable breastfeeding, then she is supported in the immediate postpartum, and she may even receive support at home after she leaves the hospital. The problem with this linear approach is that when one element fails, so does the entire model, as the next station usually does not have the pull to counteract the negative pressure exerted by the previous station, and in extreme cases of depersonalization, stations may not even be aware of what had happened in the previous process, and women in care are just "sent through the motions" of the system.

There are four especially problematic issues with this model:

*   First, there is often a lack of continuity of care, and a lack of communications, between the different elements along the "assembly line." The information and support is often unreliable, unsustainable, and conflicting.

*   Second, it ignores a holistic approach and reduces a woman to "nursing mother," with breastfeeding as the only goal, neglecting the wholeness of the person receiving attention and support.

*   Third, the near-magical harmony that must exist between all elements for the assembly line to work is simply unrealistic. When one or more elements becomes conflicting with each other, it adds duress to the family, and the centrality of breastfeeding in their lives become accentuated, instead of living

breastfeeding as an expansion in the life of the mother and the family.

- And fourth, and possibly most important, it leaves out the mother's story as the leader of the line.

To effectively help women breastfeed, health care professionals, policy makers, and advocates must first become "communicating vessels" that bring together a woman's story and help her craft a breast-feeding plan that attends all her needs. The assembly-line process does exactly the opposite, and breastfeeding becomes even more time-con-suming, stressful, and draining for women already struggling to feed their babies at the breast.

The idea of applying a V-formation approach was first brought to my attention by Human Milk for Human Babies Oregon adminis-trator, Leah Callahan, who was applying it to rotating roles as needed in grassroots efforts, and to prevent volunteers burnout. In this model, breastfeeding support, health care, milk banking, and informed milk sharing are dynamic tools that can accompany mother and baby throughout the lactation years, allowing them to surpass challenges as they arise and to accomplish a varied array of breastfeeding, personal, and emotional needs. It also incorporates the mother's other social and emotional needs and accounts for unexpected situations and challenges concerning those needs. Many migratory birds fly in a V-formation. The leader of the formation does not lead the flock, but it is one of the birds that has the most energy, allowing the birds behind it to use less energy, and enabling the flock to achieve its goal. The birds at the end also work the hardest, generating a wind of energy between themselves and the lead bird. The placement in the forma-tion is dynamic, and births rotate according to their needs. Based on this V-formation, I have envisioned a holistic, dynamic support model to support breastfeeding mothers, and milk sharing recipi-ents, which places tools along the formation that fits the particular woman's circumstances, desires, and expectations. One of the lines of the V corresponds to the biological needs involved in accomplishing the breastfeeding goal. The other corresponds to the social elements that will make this goal achievable, while also enabling the mother to pursue her career and meet other social goals and emotional needs. The placement of each tool in the formation is personalized to each individual case. In this model, milk sharing is always present, whether as a lead, supportive, or fallback role.

This model is entirely based on the story of the mother and her needs and desire as whole person, as well as a larger society, where other policies and regulations are as relevant for personal fulfillment, not just as a breastfeeding mother.

There are many challenges in the application of this model. Some of those challenges are shared by the female population, in general, by the lack of policies in accommodating the needs of womanhood in work, and even social spaces. Other challenges are the same, present for all breastfeeding mothers: lack of access to quality breastfeeding support, mainly. But several challenges are specific to milk sharing:

- **Lack of knowledge about milk sharing families.** While warnings against milk sharing by health officials and professionals are abundant, the voice of milk sharing families is missing in the dialogue. Milk sharing families have gone to extraordinary lengths to provide human milk for their children. Their stories have the potential of providing extraordinary insight about the flaws of the health care system, obstacles to breastfeeding, and safety measures needed to engage in safe milk sharing. It is imperative that we create spaces to listen to the narratives of milk sharing families, and that a body of evidence-based research is created to support families in their choices.

- **Lack of support from health professionals**. Due to the strong discouragement from health officials, understandably, health professionals do not provide support for milk- sharing families, leaving this task in the hands of families. Although milk sharing carries much less risk than artificial milk, it is not an activity without risk, and health professionals could very easily reduce risk considerably with tools at their reach. Even with the right support, it is very likely that a good number of milk-sharing families would find milk sharing to be a tool, and not a long-term decision, which may happen as a direct result of not being accompanied in their journeys by health professionals.

- **Lack of regulations**. It is common in the milk-sharing community to hear aversion to any legal regulation towards milk sharing, as women's bodies are the subject of political oppression, and human milk is an extension of their bodies. Further intrusion is not particularly welcomed. However, a complete void of regulations results in only families with a certain set of skills and tools being able to resort to milk sharing. The lack of regulation creates a socioeconomic disparity, blocking underprivileged populations from access to alternatives to artificial milk. Even worse, this aversion to regulations can result in the allocation of public resources in ill-informed legislation, such as the Bill NJA3702, recently introduced in the legislature of New Jersey, to create a campaign to raise awareness about the risks of milk sharing, leaving aside all its benefits, and a risk-comparative analysis of milk sharing vs. artificial milk, which interferes with the personal agency of families. Guidelines for safe milk sharing may give health professionals the confidence to support milk-sharing families, and democratize milk sharing.

- **Relationship with milk banks**. The relationship between milk-sharing networks and milk-sharing banks is very unfortunate. The deep sense of competition expressed by milk banks, which translates in a discourse about risks, and the need for extensive screening and pasteurization of human milk, plays right into the mainstream narrative that the bodies of women, and their product, are risky, and even "dirty." This negative message about women's bodies directly impacts their likelihood of recruiting donors, as donors are generous women making an effort of love, and want the creation of their body to be celebrated, and not offended. There are deeper implications in the discourse that suggest that women may unknowingly be feeding unsafe milk to their infants, which can also be perceived as offensive, and drive donors away from milk banking. If milk banks and milk-sharing networks came together, it is much more likely that more donor milk would be transferred to milk banks, which fulfill a vital role in the health of babies and infants. Likewise, the legitimacy of milk banks could help advance milk sharing as a valid choice about infant feeding, and safer than artificial milk.

CHAPTER 31

"One-Quarter Cow and Three-Quarters Devil"

The Use and Abuse of Wet Nurses in U.S. History

Jacqueline H. Wolf

The practice of wet nursing has differed dramatically over time from country to country, and across eras and among regions within countries. In no other country did infant-feeding habits vary more starkly by region than in Germany, where breastfeeding was least common in Southern and Eastern Bavaria and Bohemia, and most common in Northern and Western Bavaria, Baden, and Hessen. In some of the areas where German women practiced *nichtstillen* (never breastfeeding), they fed their babies pap (some combination of meat or rice broth, cows' milk, sugar, and water). In those areas, residents openly threatened and ridiculed breastfeeding mothers. In Hamburg, rather than pap-feeding, wet nursing was common. Indeed, wet nursing was so prevalent there that in the 18th century, when the city housed a population of only 90,000, 5,000 wet nurses lived in the homes of the merchants, artisans, and wealthy who hired them (Kintner, 1985; Lindemann, 1981).

In England, wet nurses did not live in their employers' homes. Instead, well-to-do mothers "placed out" babies to live with wet nurses, a custom that English colonists eventually brought to colonial

North America (Campbell, 1989; McLaren, 1979). In France, hiring a wet nurse was such a common practice among all classes that in the 18th century, Paris and Lyon were, literally, cities without babies. Working-class urban families sent their infants to even poorer women in the French countryside. So many women worked as wet nurses that the government regulated the occupation. The practice was so culturally engrained, that the Bureau of Wet Nurses was one of the few institutions to survive the French Revolution (Lehning, 1982; Sussman, 1982; Sherwood, 2010).

Unlike in France, where the practice was public and pervasive, wet nursing in the United States was a hidden, unregulated practice, and so the precise extent of the use of wet nurses there is unknown. Historians do know, however, that by the 19th century, babies were no longer "placed out" to live in wet nurses' homes. Rather, wet nurses lived with the families who hired them. These families were largely well-to-do—accustomed to supervising multiple servants. In order to procure a wet nurse, wealthy urbanites customarily dispatched the family doctor to find one. For the physicians who cared for sick infants, the task appeared to be central to their duties. Families also ran occasional ads in newspapers to procure a wet nurse (Golden, 1996; Wolf, 2001).

Doctors' writings, help wanted ads in newspapers, and wealthy women's diaries and letters to magazines, indicate that wet nurses were employed in the United States into the first decades 20th century. Detailed records of their day-to-day lives, however, are scant. There are no photographs of wet nurses. Their names are unknown. As impoverished and desperate women, they had no voice. Their employers, however, did leave some stories about the experience of wet nursing from their perspective. Their descriptions paint a disquieting picture of the institution.

The American women who hired wet nurses were vague about why. Diary entries and personal letters written to family members implied that an inability to lactate was so common among upper-class women that explanations were necessary. Physicians offered their own reasons. Isaac Abt, a prominent Chicago pediatrician, complained that women who hired wet nurses were capable of breastfeeding, but disliked the activity because it prevented them from socializing (Abt, 1944). Other doctors explained that wealthy women feared that lactation would impair their health by sapping their strength, so they hired women of supposedly hardier stock to nurse their babies (Golden, 1996; Wolf, 2001).

The families who employed wet nurses, and the doctors who searched for them, harbored stereotypical notions of who made the best and worst wet nurses. One doctor advised, "Italians and southern Negroes, when removed from their home environment secrete a milk poor in quality." Others claimed that wet nurses from Northern and Central Europe, and of Slavic descent "offer[ed] the ideal material." Irish and German immigrants were said to produce abundant milk, while American-born women were thought to be especially inadequate wet nurses due to their "flat and narrow chests" (Hess, 1928; Allen, 1889).

A wet nurse was not always the first choice of a wealthy mother. Some were heartbroken by their inability to breastfeed. Josephine Laflin, for example, a Chicago mother and the wife of a prominent Chicago architect, complained that Miss Kunz, the woman she hired to care for her newborn second son in 1898, "was most scientific and watchful in her care of baby and me, but her face was like marble, her demeanor like an iceberg, and she was as devoid of sympathy as a machine. She kept baby in another room day and night, would scarcely allow me to look at him, and never spoke of him." According to Laflin's diary, she had "hoped with all [...] [her] heart [...] to nurse baby and everything seemed propitious at first," but she soon she was sorely disappointed (Laflin Family papers).

Having relegated the care of her son to a nurse who intimidated her, Laflin's distress was probably inevitable. The nurse banned her from the nursery, precluding any chances of building an adequate milk supply. Miss Kunz proceeded to buy modified cows' milk for the baby through the local Walker-Gordon milk laboratory (Laflin Family papers). "Milk laboratories" were a burgeoning "scientific" urban industry in the late 19th-century United States. Chemists at the lab "humanized" cows' milk according to the complicated written prescriptions devised for each baby by their pediatrician (Wolf, 2001).

Although initially heartsick about her inability to breastfeed, bottle-feeding freed Laflin. Suddenly able to travel with her husband from Chicago to New York to greet her in-laws when they returned from an extended European vacation, Laflin wrote in her diary, "I gave them a genuine surprise for they never thought of my being able to leave Baby so soon" (Laflin Family papers). As evidenced by her in-laws great surprise, hiring a wet nurse, while not unusual, was not a universal custom among upper-class American women in the late 19th century.

While the Walker-Gordon concoction agreed with Laflin's baby, most women in Laflin's position would have eventually hired a wet nurse because cows' milk during that era often sickened babies. Through the 19th century, and for at least two decades into the 20th, cows' milk was not pasteurized. It was not refrigerated during shipping. The adulteration of milk was common. In the absence of any laws regulating the dairy industry, milk-borne disease was rampant. Yet cows' milk feeding was so common, that in 1900, 13 percent of infants did not live to see their first birthday. More than half the dead died of infant diarrhea, commonly known as "summer complaint," due to its seasonal occurrence. Pediatricians and public health officials attributed the high death rate from diarrhea to artificial feeding (Wolf, 2001).

Wet nurses rescued some of these infants from the edge of death. Yet despite the role they played in wealthy families, the lives of wet nurses stood in stark contrast to the lives of their privileged employers.

As single mothers, wet nurses were shunned. Possibly widowed, but most often abandoned by the father of their child and their families, they were usually homeless before finding employment. The most disturbing indication of their desperation was the requirement that, in order to work as a wet nurse in the late 19th century U.S., they had to abandon their own baby. Ads for wet nurses customarily read "Wanted: Wet Nurse WITHOUT a baby." Wealthy families were adamant—they did not want any attention diverted from their own infant. They forced the wet nurses they hired to place their own babies in foundling homes, where caretakers fed them cows' milk. The infant death rate in foundling homes was appalling—approaching 100 percent. When a woman provided her milk to save the life of a wealthy woman's baby in exchange for a temporary roof over her head, she was essentially forced to sacrifice the life of her own baby (Wolf, 2001).

The story of one woman's experience as an employer of wet nurses illustrates the horrifying dilemma wet nurses faced. In a letter to *Babyhood* magazine in 1886, Fanny B. Workman described her travails (Workman, 1886). Workman was the wife of a physician, and the daughter of a former Massachusetts governor. As an author and explorer who set world records in mountain climbing, she eventually became a woman of some renown (Golden, 1996). Although Workman clearly wrote the letter to *Babyhood* in order to air her perspective on the difficulties faced by the employers of wet nurses, her letter vividly illustrates the typical experience of a wet nurse. That was not her intent. As the product of an unashamedly class-based, racist, nativist society, she wrote the letter seeking sympathy for herself.

According to Workman, her bottle-fed daughter fell ill soon after birth. Workman immediately summoned two doctors who both suggested hiring a wet nurse. In despair, Workman anticipated "an end of all peace in the household" (Workman, 1886). Her dismay was a characteristic response—wet nurses were deemed the most troublesome of household employees.

Workman hired "a simple, unintelligent-looking Irish girl" who, at Workman's insistence, "placed out" her own baby before starting the job. Workman then devoted an entire week "to the renovation of the person of the Irish Mary, whom it was necessary to clothe anew from head to foot" (Workman, 1886). Eventually satisfied with the wet nurses' appearance, Workman was still troubled; "If only the look of intelligence were not wanting!" She expanded on her list of grievances. The wet nurse was slow to get out of the way of oncoming carriages when she took Workman's baby for a walk. When the nurse carried the infant, "the child's head hung over her arm and vibrated like a pendulum." The wet nurse consumed all the foods that Workman forbade her—tea, ice water, and pickles—lest they spoil her milk. Workman was forced to fire the cook, a "weak minded individual" (Workman, 1886), who provided the sneaky wet nurse with the foods.

The situation worsened. After a few weeks in the Workman household, the wet nurse learned that her own baby had taken ill and she wanted to go to her immediately. To persuade her to stay, Workman arranged for the infant to be cared for at a nearby farmhouse at Workman's expense. But after two weeks, the farmer's wife declared the baby to be too much work. When the wet nurse learned that her baby had to be placed elsewhere, she became so distraught that "her milk had a decidedly bad effect on her charge." Workman fired her (Workman, 1886).

Workman quickly found another wet nurse who was "decidedly unattractive, with a face of most heavy, unintelligent mould." To make matters worse, she arrived with her own baby in her arms. Workman immediately ordered her to place the baby out if she wanted the job. The wet nurse complied. Two weeks later, the nurse received a telegram informing her of her own baby's death. Frantic with grief, she prepared to attend her baby's funeral. Workman was furious, saying "After an hour or two spent in argument I prevailed upon her NOT to go to the funeral. How I made her see that it could in no way *benefit* her to go, and might kill *my* child, I do not know. But finally she did see it all" (Workman, 1886).

This did not end Workman's problems, however. After the death of her child, the wet nurse was not so easily ordered about. She became "very unruly and obstinate" and, like the first wet nurse, ate foods that did not agree with Workman's baby. Workman fired her. Rather than hire a third wet nurse, Workman offered her baby Mellin's Food "with perfect success." Workman concluded the letter by observing that "the milk of the gentle cow has the advantage over that of the wet nurse—it is not affected by indulgence in peanuts, cucumbers, and ice cream" (Workman, 1886).

Workman refused to admit that she owed her daughter's life to the efforts of wet nurses. She never acknowledged that her daughter's wet nurses had sacrificed the health of their own infants in order to sustain the health and life of Workman's baby. To the contrary, Workman expressed outrage that women who she deemed to be irresponsible, ignorant, uncouth, and sinful had to handle her baby at all. Workman exhibited no understanding of, or sympathy, for the plight of her baby's wet nurses. She steadfastly refused to recognize the little that she did share with the two women: motherhood.

Workman was hardly alone in her attitude. Other wealthy mothers shared Workman's indignation, writing to *Babyhood* to commiserate with her. One mother asked, "How can any mother dare [...] risk [...] the effect upon her child of a wet nurse in whose family some terrible disease may be hereditary, or, what is worse than disease or death, who is an immoral woman?" (Nursery Problems, 1886). Many doctors shared this view. As one Chicago doctor wrote in 1896: "a good wet nurse" may benefit her charge more than artificial food but employers had to be prepared to face the reality that "a wet nurse is one-quarter cow and three-quarters devil" (Churchill, 1896).

The wet nurses, forced to trade their babies' lives for employment, received no job security in return. One doctor reported that the mother of one infant hired 13 wet nurses in 14 days (Rotch, 1896). Although that was extreme, it was not unusual for one infant to be fed by half a dozen or more different women within two years.

By the early 20th century, fewer women were willing to wet nurse for an insecure, miserable living, and doctors, medical charities, and municipalities devised other solutions to solve the problems posed by the dearth of human milk. Articles appeared in women's magazines suggesting that women with a "superabundance" of milk share with women unable to nurse (Wolf, 2001). In the 1910s, some cities, most notably Boston, opened Wet Nurse Bureaus. These bureaus screened women, and then issued them certificates of health, effectively acting as wet-nurse employment agencies. Women who worked for Wet Nurse Bureaus were allowed to keep their babies with them (Bedinger, 1915; Talbot, 1911). By then, the high death rate among wet nurses' babies had become a scandal in the medical community. Pediatricians, in particular, were well aware of the problem; Chicago pediatrician Isaac Abt wrote of it extensively in his autobiography (Abt, 1944). If an employer seeking to hire a wet nurse through a bureau balked at allowing that wet nurse to bring her own baby with her, the bureau denied the would-be employer the employee (Golden, 1996; Wolf, 2001). Rather than a bureau, New York City pursued a more macabre route. Workers for the city's infant welfare program perused incoming death certificates for stillbirths. When they found one, a worker was immediately dispatched to ask if the dead infant's mother would be willing to work as a wet nurse (Abstract, 1917).

By the 1910s, doctors were urging hospitals to employ live-in wet nurses whose babies lived with them on site. There, they supplied milk largely to premature infants. In 1922, the Sarah Morris Children's Hospital in Chicago opened the largest premature infant station in the country, where pediatricians and nurses determined that the keys to the survival of premature babies were: 1) maintenance of body temperature, 2) prevention of infection, and 3) consumption of human milk. If a mother did not supply her premature infant with milk, then one of the hospital's resident wet nurses did. Wet nurses' hospital jobs, although not as precarious as they had been in private homes, were nevertheless temporary. When their own babies were 8 months old, wet nurses were fired due to their aged milk. Still desperately poor, few had a home to go to after leaving the hospital (Michael Reese Hospital Papers).

The number of women working as wet nurses in the United States waned slowly in proportion to the growing safety of artificial food. The passage of pure food laws requiring that milk be pasteurized before sale, refrigerated during shipping, and sealed in individual bottles, was instrumental in ending the practice of wet-nursing by the 1920s. Artificial feeding had become safer, so wet nurses were no longer needed (Wolf, 2001).

Although the institution of wet nursing was intended to save the lives of select infants and preserve the health of their mothers, wet nursing arguably contributed to more ill health and death among mothers and babies than any other practice in the countries where the custom was common. Lactation is nature's way of spacing human pregnancies. The mothers who hired strangers to suckle their children found themselves perpetually pregnant during their childbearing years, contributing to their own ill health and premature deaths. Infants fared far worse. The infants sent to wet nurses' homes died in much higher numbers than the infants who remained with their mothers, whether they were maternally breastfed, wet-nursed, or artificially fed. When employers hired live-in wet nurses, they customarily forced those employees to board their own infants in foundling homes, where those babies were warehoused. Fed artificially and largely neglected, death rates among wet nurses' infants exceeded 90 percent. The babies of impoverished women were effectively sacrificed so the babies of wealthy women could live. Across time and space, the institution of wet nursing debilitated many more mothers than it strengthened, and killed many more infants than it saved.

References

Abt, I. (1944). *Baby doctor.* New York: Whittlesey House.

Bedinger, G, R. (1915). The wet nurse directory of Boston. *Transactions of the Annual Meeting of the American Association for the Study and Prevention of Infant Mortality, 252-254.*

Campbell, L. (1989). Wet-nurses in early modern England: Some evidence from the Townshend archive. *Medical History, 33*, 360-370.

Churchill, F.S. (1896). Infant feeding. *Chicago Medical Recorder, 10*, 102-114.

Golden, J. (1996). A social history of wet nursing in America: From breast to bottle. Cambridge: Cambridge University Press.

Hess, J. (1928). *Feeding and nutritional disorders in infancy and childhood.* Philadelphia: F. A. Davis Co.

Kintner, H.J. (1985). Trends and regional differences in breastfeeding in Germany from 1871 to 1937. *Journal of Family History, 10*, 163-182.

Laflin Family papers. (n.d.). *Chicago History Museum Archives.* Chicago, IL.

Lehning, J.R. (1982). Family life and wetnursing in a French village. *Journal of Interdisciplinary History, 12*, 645-656.

Lindemann, M. (1981). Love for hire: The regulation of the wet-nursing business in eighteenth-century Hamburg. *Journal of Family History, 5*, 379-395.

McLaren, D. (1979). Nature's contraceptive: Wet-nursing and prolonged lactation: The case of Chesham, Buckinghamshire, 1578-1601. *Medical History, 23*, 426-441.

Michael Reese Hospital Papers. *Chicago Jewish Archives.* Chicago, IL: Spertus College.

Nursery Problems. (1886). *Babyhood*, 245-246.

Rotch, T.M. (1896). *Pediatrics: The hygienic and medical treatment of children.* Philadelphia: J. B. Lippincott Company.

Sherwood, J. (2010). *Infection of the innocents: Wet nurses, infants, and syphilis in France, 1780-1900.* Montreal: McGill-Queens University Press.

Sussman, G.D. (1982). *Selling mothers' milk: The wet-nursing business in France 1715-1915*. Urbana: University of Illinois Press.

Talbot, F.B. (1911). A directory for wet-nurses: Its experiences for twelve months. *Journal of the American Medical Association, 56*, 1715-1717.

Wolf, J.H. (2001). *Don't kill your baby: Public health and the decline of breastfeeding in the 19th and 20th centuries*. Columbus, OH: Ohio State University Press.

Workman, F. (1886). Letter to the Mother's Parliament. *Babyhood, 2*, 142-144.

CHAPTER 32

Effect of Maternal Employment on Infant Feeding Practices in Southwestern Nigeria

Beatrice Olubukola Ogunba

Abstract

The study investigated the effect of maternal employment on breastfeeding and childcare practices of mothers in Southwestern Nigeria. Information was collected on maternal socioeconomic characteristics, care, and feeding practices of 450 mothers selected by simple random sampling procedure from both urban and rural communities. Results revealed that the sampled mothers (46.9%) spent more than 8 hours at work and 62.7% worked outside their homes. Children received water (61.1%) as pre-lacteal feeds, and only 24% were exclusively breastfed. The mean number of breastfeeds per day was 9.7±3.9, and 37.3% introduced complementary foods at 6 months, while 68.6% terminated breastfeeding between 13 to 18 months.

Mothers who worked outside their home, in offices and factories, practiced exclusive breastfeeding, compared to those that are not working or work at home. About 58.2% of the children studied were stunted, 23.8% were wasted, and 7.8% were underweight. A significant association was found between maternal place of employment. It is strongly associated with the timing of introduction of complementary foods ($p<0.02$) and number of snack consumed/day ($p<0.03$). The study concluded that maternal place of work can positively influence the adoption of appropriate infant-feeding practice. It was, therefore, recommended that working mothers should receive more support in the workplace for them to practice appropriate feeding practices.

Introduction

In Nigeria, mothers rarely follow the appropriate infant-feeding recommendations. Infants are given pre-lacteal feeds, such as water to "welcome the child to the world," while others received concoctions to "wash off all the dirt accumulated in the stomach of the new born after delivery." Glucose is one of the pre-lacteal feeds usually given to infants as mothers await the letdown of human milk from the mammary gland. Pre-lacteal feeding is a major barrier to exclusive breastfeeding (Akuse & Obinya 2002; Khanal, **Adhikari, Sauer, & Zhao, 2013).** Only about 13% of children under 6 months are exclusively breastfed, and 87% of Nigerian infants under 6 months receive complementary liquids or foods (Nigerian Demographic and Health Survey, 2008). These inappropriate feeding behaviors are an important determinant of malnutrition (Dili, 2010).

Human milk has nutritional, immunological, biochemical, anti-allergic, anti-infective, intellectual, developmental, psychological, psychosocial, economic, and environmental benefits for the mother and her infant (Earle, 2002; Lawrence et al., 2003). Majority of the infants in Nigeria are introduced to cereal-based complementary foods well before the recommended 6 months age, for the introduction of "safe and nutritionally adequate" complementary foods or, in rare instances, do not receive these until the 2nd year (Onyango, 2003). In order to understand the effect of maternal employment on feeding practices, this paper examined infant feeding practices *vis-à-vis* maternal employment in Southwestern Nigeria.

Method

The study was conducted in Osun State Southwestern, Nigeria. A multi-stage, random sampling procedure was employed. Only 450 mothers of children between the ages of 0 to 24 months were selected. Information was sought with the use of structured interview schedule on the socioeconomic characteristics of mothers and feeding practices. Anthropometric measurements were taken and converted to z-scores to determine nutritional status. Data were analyzed with the SPSS package 16.0 and Nutrisurvey.

Results

Maternal Characteristics

The majority (48.2%) of mothers were aged 20 to 29, and 46.7% worked more than 8 hours a day. Only 10.4 percent were not employed. Twenty-six point nine percent worked at home, 25.3% worked in the market place, and 37.4% worked in an office or shop. Only 6.7% of children of mothers working outside the home were cared for in the crèches during working hours. Others were in the daycare centers (31.8%), while 61.5% were at home with other caregivers (See Table 1).

Infant and Young Child Feeding Practices

Results on Table 2 reveal that children received pre-lacteal feeding, though 86.4% of mothers initiated breastfeeding within 6 hours of birth. The mean and standard deviation number of breastfeeds/day was 9.7 ± 3.9. Only 23.9% of children were exclusively breastfed. The mean age of introduction of complementary feeding was 4.4 ± 2.2 and mean duration of breastfeeding was 11.9 ± 7.9. Only 21.3% of mothers breastfed their children after the children attained the age of 18 months. The mean number of complementary foods/day was 2.7 ± 1.4 while that of snacks was 1.7 ± 0.9 (See Table 2).

Place of Employment and Feeding Practices

The patterns of breastfeeding followed the same pattern, irrespective of the place of maternal employment. The number of breastfeeds/day was, however, higher for mothers working in factories or offices. The timing of the introduction of complementary foods ($p<0.02$), and number of snack consumed/day ($p<0.03$), were significant with the place of employment of mothers (See Table 3).

Discussion

Young child feeding practices in Nigeria rarely follow the recommendation of major health organizations. Children received pre-lacteal feedings, such as water, glucose, and infant formula. This is corroborated by Lakati et al, (2010) study in Kenya of the prevalence of 26.8% pre-lacteal feeds: the most common were infant formula and glucose solution. Pre-lacteal feeds have lesser nutrient and immunological value, and are often likely to introduce contaminants (Laroia & Sharma, 2006). Though most mothers initiated breastfeeding on time, infants received less breastfeedings per day, as children received other liquids, especially infant formula, apart from human milk. Mothers in the urban communities practice exclusive breastfeeding more than their rural counterparts.

Complementary foods were introduced before 6 months, at an average of 4.4 years ± 2.2. This is also revealed in Sellen (2001), study with an average age of 4.5 years ± 6.0. Most mothers do not breastfeed up until the age of 2 years, as breastfeeding was terminated between 12 to 18 months. Mothers in the rural areas, however, had longer duration of breastfeeding. This is probably because their children are with them most of the time, as compared to the urban communities' mothers, who have their babies in the crèche or daycare.

Mothers' place of employment may be an important factor in the choice of feeding practices. In this study, mothers who worked outside the home had better feeding practices, when compared to the non-working mothers, and those who worked at home. Mothers' workplace was related to a significant difference in the timing of the introduction of the complementary foods, and the number of snacks consumed per day. The approved maternity leave in Nigeria is for 3 months, after which the mother will have to resume working. It is noted that mothers who worked at home introduce complementary foods earlier than mothers who worked outside the home. The adoption of appropriate feeding practices, therefore, is not negatively influenced by maternal occupation and place of work. Maternal occupation influenced feeding practices positively. Mothers who worked in the offices and factories are likely to be educated, and may have been influenced in their workplaces, and gained knowledge of childcare from other nursing mothers. Maternal decisions to breastfeed are influenced by knowledge, support, and help with difficulties (Brown, Raynor, & Lee, 2011), not necessarily the place or type of job.

Conclusion

Appropriate feeding practices by mothers are influenced by maternal employment. However, the influence is not negative. Mothers should be adequately informed about correct practices and, in place of employment, should receive support both at home and in workplaces.

References

Akuse, R. M., & Obinya, E. A. (2002). Why healthcare workers give prelacteal feeds. *European Journal of Clinical Nutrition, 56*(8), 729-734.

Brown, A., Raynor, P., & Lee, M. (2011). Healthcare professionals' and mothers' perceptions of factors that influence decisions to breastfeed or formula feed infants: A comparative study. *Journal of Advanced Nursing, 67*(9), 1993-2003. doi: 10.1111/j.1365-2648.2011.05647.x.

Dili, T.-L. (2010). 2008 behavior change communication strategy for child health. *East Africa Journal of Public Health, 7*(3), 258-62.

Earle, S. (2002). Factors affecting the initiation of breast-feeding: Implications for breast-feeding promotion. *Health Promotion International,* 17, 205–214.

Khanal, V., Adhikari, M., Sauer, K., & Zhao, Y. (2013). Factors associated with the introduction of prelacteal feeds in Nepal: Findings from the Nepal Demographic and Health Survey 2011. *International Breastfeeding Journal, 8,* 9.

Lakati, A.S., Makokha, O.A., Binns, C.W., & Kombe, Y. (2010). The effect of pre-lacteal feeding on full breastfeeding in Nairobi, Kenya. *East Africa Journal of Public Health, 7*(3), 258-262.

Laroia, N., & Sharma, D. (2006). The religious and cultural bases for breastfeeding practices among the Hindus. *Breastfeeding Medicine, 1,* 94-98.

Lawrence, N., Hand, I., Haynes, D., McVeigh, T., MaeHee, K., & Ja Yoon, J. (2003). Factors influencing initiation of breastfeeding among urban women. *American Journal of Perinatology, 20,* 477–83.

Nigeria Demographic and Health Survey (NDHS). (2008). *Key Findings.* Calverton, MD: NPC and ICF Macro.

Onyango, A.W. (2003). Dietary diversity, child nutrition and health in contemporary African communities. *Review of Comparative Biochemistry & Physiology, 136,* 61–69.

Sellen, D. W. (2001). Comparison of infant feeding patterns reported for nonindustrial populations with current recommendations. *Journal of Nutrition, 31*(10), 2707-2715.

Table 1
Frequency Distribution of Maternal Characteristics

Variables	Urban (n=337)		Rural (n=113)		Total (N=450)	
	Freq.	%	Freq.	%	Freq.	%
Age of mothers (years)						
<20	4	1.2	4	2.6	8	1.8
20-29	168	49.8	49	43.4	217	48.2
30-39	143	42.4	46	40.7	189	42
40-49	19	5.6	14	12.4	33	7.3
50-59	3	0.9	1	0.2	3	0.7
Place of Employment						
Home	74	21.9	47	41.6	121	26.9
Market/Street	79	23.1	35	31.0	114	25.3
Factory/office/shop	148	43.6	19	16.8	168	37.4
Not employed	35	10.4	12	10.6	47	10.4
Usual hours worked per day						
Zero	47	13.9	9	8.0	56	12.4
1 – 8	140	31.1	44	38.9	184	40.9
>8	150	45	60	53.1	210	46.7
Hours with children						
1 -8 hours	14	4.2	3	2.7	17	3.8
9 -16 hours	92	27.3	12	10.6	104	23.1
17 - 24 hours	231	68.5	98	86.7	329	73.1
Care Alternatives						
Crèche	7	7.5	0	0.0	7	6.7
Daycare	29	31.2	4	36.4	33	31.8
Home house help	57	61.3	7	63.6	64	61.5
***Source of information on feeding practices**						
Health workers	215	64.1	67	59.3	283	62.9
Radio	157	46.6	46	40.7	203	45.1
Television	101	30.0	9	8.0	110	24.4
Older mothers	102	30.3	51	45.1	153	34.0
Friends and Neighbors	77	22.8	37	32.7	114	25.3
Bulletins	55	16.3	04	3.5	55	12.2
Magazines	51	15.1	05	4.4	60	13.3

*Multiple responses

Table 2
Infant and Young Child Feeding Practices

Feeding practices	Urban	Rural	Total
Pre-lacteal feeding %			
Water	62.9	55.8	61.1%
Concoction	27.6	53.1	34%
Glucose	35.3	22.1	32%
Infant formula	57.3	46.9	54.7%
Initiation of breastfeeding within six hours of birth %	88.7	81.4	86.4
Number of breastfeeding/day (Mean and SD)	11.1±10.6	8.1±7.3	9.7±3.9
Duration of breastfeeding (Mean and SD)	10.8±8.0	17.5±3.6	11.9±7.9
Age of introduction of complementary food(Mean and SD)	4.6±2.1	3.8±2.4	4.4±2.2
% Exclusive breastfeeding	35.0	6.6	23.9
% Ever breastfed	100	100	100
% Breastfed less than 12 months	12.9	0.0	10.1
% Breastfed up to 12-18months	67.1	73.7	68.6
% Breastfed after 18 months	20.0	26.3	21.3
Number of complementary feeding/day(Mean and SD)	2.7±1.3	2.6±1.7	2.7±1.4
Number of snack/day(Mean and SD)	1.7±0.9	1.6±0.9	1.7±0.9

Table 3

Cross-Tabulation of Place of Employment and Feeding Practices

Place of Employment	Home		Market/ Street		Factory/ Office /Shop		Not Employed		p value
	Freq.	%	Freq.	%	Freq.	%	Freq.	%	
Exclusive breast-feeding for six months									0.86
Yes (95)	26	27.3	21	22.1	37	38.9	11	11.5	
No (355)	95	26.7	93	26.1	131	36.9	36	10.1	
Number of breast-feeding/day									0.32
<8 (75)	16	21.3	18	24.0	36	48.0	5	6.6	
>8 (148)	33	22.2	33	22.2	60	40.5	22	14.8	
Introduction of complementary food									
Before 3 months (54)	20	37.0	10	18.5	18	33.3	6	11.1	0.02*
3-6 months (193)	40	20.7	53	27.4	83	43.0	17	8.8	
>6 months (70)	18	25.7	20	28.5	27	38.5	5	7.1	
Number of comple-mentary foods/day									
1-3 (191)	51	26.7	53	27.7	65	34.0	22	11.5	0.33
>3 (78)	20	25.6	21	26.9	34	43.5	3	3.8	
Number of snacks/day									
0 (30)	7	23.3	11	36.6	7	23.3	5	16.6	
1 (45)	8	17.7	13	28.8	16	35.5	8	17.7	0.03*
>1(170)	41	24.1	48	28.2	70	41.1	11	64.7	
Duration of breast-feeding									
<12 (50)	8	16.0	14	28.0	21	42.0	7	14.0	0.14
>12months (68)	17	25.0	14	20.5	24	35.2	12	17.6	

CHAPTER 33

All-Nighters: Multi-level Ecological Approaches to Supporting Breast-feeding Mothers in Higher Education

Hannah Tello

The American Public Health Association proclaims human milk is the most appropriate food for infants. The American Academy of Pediatrics refers to breastfeeding as the "normative standard for infant feeding and nutrition," and recommends that all infants be breastfed exclusively for 6 months, with breastfeeding continuing at least through the first year (American Academy of Pediatrics [AAP], 2012). Global recommendations for breastfeeding are even more expansive, with the World Health Organization recommending breastfeeding through at least the first 2 years of life (World Health Organization [WHO], 2002).

Breastfeeding offers a critical intersection of issues related to socioeconomics and health. At a community level, breastfeeding delivers significant social benefits; a 2010 report published in the official journal of the American Academy of Pediatrics found that, "if 90% of U.S. families could comply with medical recommendations to breastfeed exclusively for 6 months, the United States would save $13 billion per year, and prevent an excess 911 deaths, nearly all of which would be infants" (Bartick & Reinhold, 2010, p. e1048). At an individual level, breastfeeding results in both reduced direct costs (such as the elimination of the need to purchase infant formula), and indirect costs (such as the reduced costs of health care, particularly for the uninsured, due to fewer infant illness and hospital visits). As such, disenfranchised mothers, including single mothers, mothers of color, and mothers living below the poverty line, stand the most to gain economically from optimal breastfeeding.

These same diverse groups are also disproportionately impacted by health disparities against which breastfeeding is known to be protective. However, these same demographic groups are also consistently less likely to initiate or sustain breastfeeding. The American Academy of Pediatrics (2012) reports that breastfeeding is protective against Sudden Infant Death Syndrome (SIDS), infant mortality, otitis media (ear infections), asthma, obesity, and diabetes. For mothers, a history of breastfeeding is correlated with a reduced risk of Type 2 diabetes, as well as reduced rates of aggressive forms of breast and ovarian cancers (Ip et al., 2007). These health conditions are differently distributed across ethnic and socioeconomic groups: morbidity and mortality rates for these health conditions are disproportionately impact mothers of color, impoverished mothers, and mothers with low educational attainment.

Addressing health disparities through breastfeeding promotion cannot be disentangled from broader discussions about wealth and poverty. Women living in poverty are more likely to be non-white, single, and of low educational attainment. Economic and social policy strategies to reduce health disparities in these populations often address the needs of this severely disenfranchised group have increasingly focused on access to immediate, low-skill employment, despite the fact that studies demonstrate that this is an unreliable and unsustainable pathway out of poverty, instead offering only temporary or limited relief (Wilson, 2011).

Increasingly, researchers and policymakers have recognized that access to higher education is a more impactful, and more sustainable, approach to long-term financial stability, particularly for single mothers and other parents (Ames, Lowe, Dowd, Liberman, & Young-blood, 2013). Impoverished and single mothers have responded in kind to this shift from immediate employment to longer-term educational attainment. In the past 20 years, enrollment of single parents in college has doubled, and significantly more single mothers are enrolling compared to single fathers (17% of all undergraduates compared to 8% respectively) (U.S. Department of Education, 2002).

Educational researchers and public health researchers have yet to substantially collaborate on the potential intersections between breast-feeding and education as paired strategies to create pathways out of poverty for diverse women. As such, women in poverty, particularly single mothers, are often poised at a challenging, if not impossible, apex of decision-making. Though enrollment in 4-year institutions is increasingly becoming not only an accessible option for upward economic mobility, but the only one that demonstrates sustainable success, the lack of progressive and proactive university and commu-nity-level policies to support women's continued efforts to breastfeed often force mothers to choose one or the other: the economic (and therefore, health) benefits of education, or the economic (and there-fore, health) benefits of breastfeeding.

The current project situates the University of Massachusetts, Lowell as a model for the development of breastfeeding-friendly Univer-sity and community policies as a strategy to unite educational and public health approaches to reducing health disparities, and creating sustainable pathways out of poverty. The risks of health disparities are particularly critical in Lowell, where 6.8 percent of the population is Black, 42 percent speak a language other than English, 24 percent is foreign-born, and 17.6 percent live below the federal poverty line (U.S. Census Bureau, 2013). The population of young, single parents, partic-ularly mothers, in Lowell is one of the highest in the state. The latest data set indicates that Lowell has the 8th highest teen birth rate in the state, with 44.7 births per every 1000 teenage women, compared to the state average of 17.1 births (*Massachusetts Births,* 2013). Nearly 67% of

Lowell's impoverished families are headed by single women (Lowell Massachusetts Poverty Rate Data, 2009). Increasingly, these single mothers are pursuing higher education, oftentimes out of necessity. In 2005, the estimated required annual income to support two dependent children in Massachusetts was $65,880, a wage nearly impossible to obtain with less than a 4-year degree (Ames et al., 2013).

The current project utilized two sets of data collected through survey research. The first set of data was collected exclusively from parenting students at UMass, Lowell, and included both demographic information and satisfaction information regarding their experience as parenting students. The second set of data was collected from faculty, staff, and students at UMass, Lowell who breastfed or pumped milk for their children while working or studying at the university.

Data from these two studies yielded important results concerning the types of resources that are most lacking, and most valuable, to parenting and breastfeeding students, faculty, and staff. Preliminary results indicated that an overwhelming number of students' parents were unsatisfied with the quality of, and access to, their on-campus resources. Ninety-one percent of participants either disagreed, or strongly disagreed, that they understood the types of services available to them. Eighty-six percent disagreed, or strongly disagreed, that they would know who to talk to if they needed help with school-life balance. Only 11.9% of participants believe that the University provides adequate support services to parenting students.

The poor access to, and understanding of, relevant resources were reiterated in the breastfeeding research. Ninety-percent of participants indicated that they were unaware of the available University resources for breastfeeding mothers. Ninety-two percent disagreed, or strongly disagreed, that finding information about resources related to breastfeeding was easy. Even more importantly, 46% of participants agreed that their involvement with the University directly interfered with their breastfeeding goals. Students and staff were more likely to indicate that their University involvement served as a barrier to their breastfeeding goals than were the faculty.

Results from these projects indicate the need to think ecologically about interventions. Though many interventions and promotional activities related to health behaviors, like breastfeeding, are focused at the individual level (for example, on building self-efficacy or breastfeeding knowledge), these results suggest that institutional changes are also critical, particularly for women who are less likely to have high levels of health-seeking behaviors, such as low-income or immigrant mothers.

Based on feedback from participants, the next phase of this project will focus on the design and presentation of both policy and infrastructure recommendations to be implemented at the University. Participants were asked to prioritize several resources in the order of how helpful they would be. In order, the following recommendations regarding support for breastfeeding mothers will be made.

1. Multiple, private, secure locations (other than a bathroom) equipped with a comfortable chair and electrical outlet for expressing human milk, or feeding a child.

2. Protected, regular breaks for students, faculty, and staff for expressing human milk or breastfeeding their children.

3. An official, written University policy for the rights and reasonable accommodations of breastfeeding mothers on campus.

4. A page on the website with information about on-campus resources and campus breastfeeding, and pumping policies.

5. A dedicated lactation liaison at the University Health Center.

6. On-site prenatal and breastfeeding education workshops.

7. A University organization for breastfeeding mothers.

8. A page on the website with information and referrals for off-campus resources for breastfeeding mothers.

9. Subsidized breast pumps.

Similar, generalized recommendations for all parenting students will also be recommended, with additional recommendations for creative solutions to childcare (on-site childcare is a very long-term project, but creative solutions to assist mothers immediately are also necessary). The next phase of this project includes the development of a strategic plan for implementation of these recommendations, as well as the development of a system for tracking the impact of transparent, comprehensive breastfeeding- and parent-friendly policies, particularly for mothers of color, single mothers, and mothers living below the poverty line.

References

American Academy of Pediatrics. (2012). Breastfeeding and the use of human milk. *Pediatrics, 129*(3), e827-e841. doi:10.1542/peds.2011-3552

Ames, M., Lowe, J., Dowd, K., Liberman, R., & Youngblood, D. (2013). *Massachusetts Economic Independence Index 2013.* Crittendon Women's Union.

Bartick, M., & Reinhold, A. (2010). The burden of suboptimal breastfeeding in the United States:A pediatric cost analysis. *Pediatrics, 125*(5), e1048-1056. doi: 10.1542/peds.2009-1616

Ip, S., Chung, M., Raman, G., Chew, P., Magula, N., DeVine, D., Trikalinos, D., & Lau, J. (2007). *Breastfeeding and maternal and infant health outcomes in developed countries* (Evidence Report/Technology Assessment No. 153). Retrieved from the U.S. Department of Health and Human Services Agency for Healthcare Research and Quality Lowell Massachusetts Poverty Rate Data. (2009). *City data.* Retrieved from http://www.city-data.com/poverty/poverty-Lowell-Massachusetts.html

Massachusetts Births 2010. (2013). Division of Research and Epidemiology, Bureau of Health Information, Statistics, Research and Evaluation. Boston: Massachusetts Department of Public Health.

U.S. Census Bureau. (2013). *Lowell (city) quickfacts from the US census bureau.* Retrieved from http://quickfacts.census.gov/qfd/states/25/2537000.html

U.S. Department of Education, National Center for Education Statistics. (2002). *Non-traditional undergraduates* (Publication No. 2002-012). Washington, DC: US Printing Office

Wilson, K. (2011). If not welfare, then what?: How single mothers finance college post-welfare reform. *Journal of Sociology & Social Welfare, 38*(4), 51-76.

World Health Organization. (2002). *Infant and young child nutrition: global strategy on infant and young child feeding* (Policy Number A55/15). Retrieved from http://apps.who.int/gb/archive/pdf_files/WHA55/ea5515.pdf

Partnering through Narrative: Social Media and Communications

We conclude this volume with several papers addressing the real issues in partnering and communication, even within the breastfeeding and feminist communities. Social media, and other communications media, are playing an increasing role in our discourse. Here we see both the supportive and challenging aspects of narratives and media experiences as breastfeeding is becoming increasingly accepted as normative in all societies.

CHAPTER 34

Social Media and Text Messaging in Peer Support for Breastfeeding

Sarah E. DeYoung and Veronica Varela

Abstract

Social support from peers is well-known to be one of the key predictors for engaging in breastfeeding and overcoming challenges associated with nursing (Chapman, 2010). According to Chapman et al. (2010), efficacy is found to be one of the major underlying factors in boosting the effects of this peer support. There are also numerous studies about the burgeoning of resources from "new" technologies, such as the Internet, and applications on Smart Phones that may bolster rates of sustained and exclusive breastfeeding (D'Auria, 2011; Ericson et al., 2013). However, there is little research to date that establishes the relationship between peer support as it is mediated through technology tools such as the use of social media, text messaging, and forum use. We propose that there is an urgent need to address the relationship between various types of social support (emotional, informational, and instrumental), and uses of technologies (hard and soft forms: mobile phones vs. social networking or blogging). Also, further research should be conducted to address the complexities of the ways in which this support is diffused in order to identify the indirect or underlying relationships between the aforementioned variables and other factors, such as personality type, external sources of information, and access to technology for communication.

Overview and Purpose

Research on decisions for breastfeeding, barriers to breastfeeding, and sustained breastfeeding has burgeoned, especially in the last 10 to 15 years. Most of the academic publications in the area of breastfeeding are from the fields of nursing, lactation, and specific health studies. However, another sub-area of research, in which there has also been an increase in research and publication, is in social science research. Specifically, issues related to social support (Kaunonen, Hannula, & Tarkka, 2012 Mitra, Khoury, Hinton, & Carothers, 2004), stigmatization of feeding choices (Kendall-Tackett & Sugarman, 1995; Rempel, 2004), maternal emotional well-being (McDaniel, Coyne, & Holmes, 2012), and broad ecological contexts related to breastfeeding (Gallegos, Russell-Bennett, & Previte, 2011) have been main topics of interest.

We reviewed key studies using the keywords social support and breastfeeding, breastfeeding and social media, breastfeeding and technology, and media and breastfeeding. We filtered our initial findings of articles from peer-review studies published from 2000 to 2014 (N=19 articles after filtering based on these qualifications). We categorized articles according to major three major themes (social support, technology and media, or integrated topics) and then created a list of subthemes, along with study limitations. Our findings suggest that this general topic is well-studied, but lacks integration between social support research through mobile devices and Internet venues. There is especially a dearth of research regarding social support that occurs emergently, rather than through interventions or group assessments.

Literature Review

Of the topics we identified, social support seems to be a unifying theme because it is included as a crucial variable in most studies related to the sustainability and maintenance of breastfeeding. Social support is defined as "the active participation of significant others in an individual's stress management efforts" (Thoits, 1986, as cited in Moritsugu, Vera, Wong, & Duffy, 2014, p. 67). There are three main kinds of social support: instrumental (giving someone resources to achieve a goal), emotional (giving someone emotional compassion and empathy in the face of obstacles or difficulties), and informative (giving someone information about the best way to achieve a goal based on pre-discovered best practices related to the specific goal) (Moritsugu et al., 2014). Many studies show the benefit of social support, not only for the decision to breastfeed (Gallegos, Russell-Bennett, & Previte, 2011), but also the effect of social support on maternal well-being (McDaniel, Coyne, & Holmes, 2012). These studies display the effects of all three aforementioned types of support, depending on the context and process of implementation of the interventions. The populations that these interventions target range from vulnerable to privileged, and yet results suggest that social support positively impacts breastfeeding duration (Edwards, Bickmore, Jenkins, Foley, & Manjourides, 2013; Fallon, et al., 2005; Grassley, 2010).

Another area of research that is new and rapidly aggregating is the area of social media, and use of mobile devices, and of various technologies for improved and maintained breastfeeding. These studies include measurements about the effectiveness of programs, such as Text4Baby (Gazmararian, Elon, Yang, Graham, & Parker, 2013), as well as studies of online activities of nursing mothers (D'Auria, 2011; McDaniel, Coyne, & Holmes, 2012; Kaunonen, Hannula, & Tarkka, 2012; Song, West, Lundy, & Dahmen, 2012). Results from these studies suggest that the use of mobile devices, Internet social media, and other Internet-based means for gathering and disseminating information, may have a positive impact on maternal well-being, loyalty, or commitment to breastfeeding, and trouble-shooting for common problems encountered related to breastfeeding (i.e., latching, thrush, etc.). However, it remains unclear how emergent (naturally occurring on a peer-to-peer level) communication patterns occur, and how these communication patterns are impacted by external and internal factors related to the nursing mother. Internal factors would be variables, such as personality traits, intelligence, education, or demographic characteristics, whereas external factors might be categorized as the following: ease and frequency of access to mobile devices and technologies, geographic location, cultural and political settings, norms and decorum, and family structure.

Limitations of Existing Research

In a review of the 19 studies, we found some methodological limitations. For example, three of the studies did not have a control group (Gazmararian etal., 2013; McDaniel, Coyne, & Holmes, 2012; Parkinson, Russell-Bennett, & Previte, 2012). Also, low sample size was also an issue for some of the studies, which could have an adverse impact on statistical power (Shadish, Cook, & Campbell, 2002). Possibly affecting the generalizability of the research was lack of diverse population of participants. For example, one study's participant pool was composed of mostly White mothers (McDaniel, Coyne, & Holmes, 2012).

Another limitation of content was that most of the present literature focuses on the effects of face-to-face social support rather than virtual support. Though face-to-face social support was popular, much of the support came from professionals in the field, such as lactation consultants or certified nurses (Ahmed & Ouzzani, 2013; D'Auria, 2011; Edwards et al., 2013). Much of the research assesses the usefulness of the medical support (i.e., support that is available for mothers through their doctors, hospitals, and partners). The existing research on mobile support focuses on the satisfaction of the programs, as well as measures the usability of the support (Gazmararian et al., 2013) rather than the program's implications on the mother, and the sustainability of breastfeeding.

Also, most of the research about mobile support focuses on programs whose main form of communication is one way with the messages sent to the participant automatically (Gazmararian et al., 2013). There was one study that included bidirectional communication in which the participant was able to keep an online diary of her experience with breastfeeding, and had access to a lactation consultant virtually (Ahmed & Ouzzani, 2013). Also, in an intervention conducted by Edwards et al. (2013) an interactive, computer-based program offered a two-way dialogue between the mother and a "computer agent." Although this program did offer a form of bidirectional communication, the communication was not between the mother and her peer(s), and was limited in the type of information that was exchanged. Therefore, although both of these studies (Ahmed & Ouzzani, 2013; Edwards et al., 2013) had a form of bidirectional communication, we would not categorize as an assessment of peer support because the information exchange was between the mother and a health professional or computer agent (respectively).

Suggestions for Future Research

To address the methodological issues, we propose that more longitudinal and cross-sectional studies should be considered, along with the inclusion of larger, and more diverse, samples. In order to measure the effects of social support on breastfeeding behaviors, a longitudinal study would assess the long-term effects on the length of time for nursing, as well as the effects that social support can have on the mother and child's well-being. These studies could be conducted through both qualitative and quantitative data-gathering techniques.

To address the content limitations (i.e., the types of variables measured for assessing breastfeeding outcomes), we suggest that there is a need for the future to focus on implications of emergent social support that occurs through social media, and that there should be an assessment of how this social support occurs through various technological devices (frequency of use of mobile phone, home computer, tablet, or voice or video through the phone). We also suggest that the research should be designed in a way that would explore specific motivations for mothers to seek to social support, as well as why they decide to share and/or seek information (i.e., what predicts the mother to become an "information sharer" versus "information seeker?"). These predictors might include personality traits, the specific experience with breastfeeding (duration, frequency, and valence of the breastfeeding experience).

Conclusion

The ultimate goal of our suggestions is to improve the well-being of mothers and their offspring through carefully planned research in this rapidly growing area of research. Breastfeeding, social support, and the use of technologies will likely be an area of interest for many years to come, especially with the rapid advancement of innovation in social media and communication devices. Given the broad range of possibilities of directions for future research on breastfeeding and social support, we anticipate that our suggestions may be useful for a variety of disciplines and research goals.

References

Ahmed, A., & Ouzzani, M. (2013). Development and assessment of an interactive web-based breastfeeding monitoring system (LACTOR). *Maternal and Child Health Journal, 17*(5), 809-815. doi:10.1007/s10995-012-1074-z

Chapman, D. J. (2010). The costs of suboptimal breastfeeding. *Journal of Human Lactation, 26,* 338-339. doi:10.1177/0890334410378264

D'Auria, J. P. (2011). The digital age: Top breastfeeding resources. *Journal of Pediatric Health Care, 25*(4), e13-e16. doi:http://dx.doi.org.prox.lib. ncsu.edu/10.1016/j.pedhc.2011.04.001

Edwards, R. A., Bickmore, T., Jenkins, L., Foley, M., & Manjourides, J. (2013). Use of an interactive computer agent to support breastfeeding. *Maternal and Child Health Journal.* doi:10.1007/s10995-013-1222-0

Ericson, J., Eriksson, M., Hellstrom-Westas, L., Hagberg, L., Hoddinott, P., & Flacking, R. (2013). The effectiveness of proactive telephone support provided to breastfeeding mothers of preterm infants: Study protocol for a randomized controlled trial. *BMC Pediatrics, 13*(1), 73. Retrieved from http://www.biomedcentral.com/1471-2431/13/73

Fallon, A. B., Hegney, D., O'Brien, M., Brodribb, W., Crepinsek, M., & Doolan, J. (2005). An evaluation of a telephone-based postnatal support intervention for infant feeding in a regional Australian Citya. *Birth, 32*(4), 291-298. doi:10.1111/j.0730-7659.2005.00386.x

Gallegos, D., Russell-Bennett, R., & Previte, J. (2011). An innovative approach to reducing risks associated with infant feeding: The use of technology. *Journal of Nonprofit & Public Sector Marketing, 23*(4), 327-347. doi:10.1080/10495142.2011.623504

Gazmararian, J. A., Elon, L., Yang, B., Graham, M., & Parker, R. (2013). Text4baby program: An opportunity to reach underserved pregnant and postpartum women? *Maternal and Child Health Journal.* doi:10.1007/s10995-013-1258-1

Grassley, J. S. (2010). Adolescent mothers' breastfeeding social support needs. *Journal of Obstetric, Gynecologic, & Neonatal Nursing, 39*(6), 713-722. doi:10.1111/j.1552-6909.2010.01181.x

Kendall-Tackett, K.A., & Sugarman, M. (1995). The social consequences of long-term breastfeeding. *Journal of Human Lactation, 11*, 179-183. doi:10.1177/089033449501100316

Kaunonen, M., Hannula, L., & Tarkka, M. (2012). A systematic review of peer support interventions for breastfeeding. *Journal of Clinical Nursing, 21*(13-14), 1943-1954. doi:10.1111/j.1365-2702.2012.04071.x

McDaniel, B. T., Coyne, S. M., & Holmes, E. K. (2012). New mothers and media use: Associations between blogging, social networking, and maternal well-being. *Maternal and Child Health Journal, 16*(7), 1509-1517. doi:10.1007/s10995-011-0918-2

Mitra, A. K., Khoury, A. J., Hinton, A. W., & Carothers, C. (2004). Predictors of breastfeeding intention among low-income women. *Maternal & Child Health Journal, 8*(2), 65-70. Retrieved from http://

search.ebscohost.com/login.aspx?direct=true&db=a9h&AN=1295
4215&site=ehost-live&scope=site

Moritsugu, J., Vera, E., Wong, F. Y., & Duffy, K. G. (2014). *Community Psychology*. (5th Edition).Parkinson, J., Russell-Bennett, R., & Previte, J. (2012). Mum or bub? Which influences breastfeeding loyalty. *Australasian Marketing Journal (AMJ)*, *20*(1), 16-23. doi:http:// dx.doi.org.prox.lib.ncsu.edu/10.1016/j.ausmj.2011.10.010

Rempel, L. A. (2004). Factors influencing the breastfeeding decisions of long-term breastfeeders. *Journal of Human Lactation*, *20*, 306-318. doi:10.1177/0890334404266969

Shadish, W. R., Cook, T. D., & Campbell, D. T. (2002). *Experimental and quasi-experimental designs for generalized causal inference*. Boston, MA: Houghton Mifflin.

Song, F. W., West, J. E., Lundy, L., & Dahmen, N. S. (2012). Women, pregnancy, and health information online: The making of informed patients and ideal mothers. *Gender & Society, 26*(5), 773-798. doi:10.1177/0891243212446336

Comparisons of Social Representations of Breastfeeding in Social Advertising in Montréal

Chantal Bayard

Overview

In Quebec, the change in standard infant feeding is well underway. For most women, breastfeeding is recognized as the preferred feeding mode. According to the *2011 to 2012 Canadian Community Health Survey*, 89% of Quebecers have initiated breastfeeding at birth in 2011 to 2012, which proves a significant increase compared to 2003 (76%), and catching the Canadian average (89.4%) (*Statistiques Canada*, 2013). However, although in progress, the rate of exclusive breastfeeding up to 6 months in Quebec is 19%, which puts it below the national average (26%). Over the past 15 years, the Quebec government has repeatedly taken a stand for the promotion, protection, and support of breastfeeding (*Ministère de la santé*, 1997, 2001, 2003, 2008, 2010).

Each year, the World Breastfeeding Week remains a special time for the government, and breastfeeding support groups, to inform and educate women on breastfeeding. In this context, the Montreal's Department of Public Health usually chose that moment to join forces. Although active for several years in the field, this conference will focus on campaigns released in the last two years. In 2012, the Montreal's Department of Public Health launched a campaign to promote breastfeeding with the following slogan: "Breastfeeding is glamorous" (*Agence de la santé*, 2012). It featured an actress, well-known to the general public, breastfeeding her 9-month-old daughter, sitting on a chair, showing off her legs, and dressed in a sexy way. She looked us straight in the eye, and said, "I breastfeed too." The ad got significant visibility in Quebec, and stirred much criticism. This year, the same organization launched a much less conspicuous ad, focusing on topics, such as the benefits of breastfeeding, and the importance of confidence and support (*Agence de la santé*, 2014). This time around, the same actress appears in a video wearing a pink cardigan on a white background. One woman. Two different performances. Two campaigns of variable visibility. What does this tell us about Quebec society?

Method

My analysis will focus on the social representations conveyed in the promotional materials on breastfeeding developed under both campaigns launched by the Montreal's Department of Public Health. My theoretical framework is based on the work on social representations of Denise Jodelet (2003a-b). For purposes of analysis, two images, featuring Mahée Payment, a French Quebec actress and business woman well-known to the general public, were selected. The first, published in 2012, is a poster of the actress breastfeeding her 9-month-old daughter, looking the public straight in the eye. The second, published in 2013, is a still image of the actress breastfeeding and speaking in a video produced, and made available online, by Montreal's Department of Public Health. I will add to these images, the analysis of newspapers articles, and television interviews concerning the development of the 2012 campaign "Breastfeeding is Glamorous."

Results

To date, analysis of selected promotional material reveals that the Department of Public Health offers, from one year to another, opposing representations of women and mothers in their campaign. The image built in 2012 is close to commercial advertising, and seeks, in this context, to "sell" breastfeeding in putting forward the representation of a sexualized mother. In this ad, the actress portrays the "celebrity body," and the "hot mama," by focusing on the sexual power of women's bodies. In the second campaign, launched in 2013, the image puts forward the "everyday mom." Thus, the actress performs the "girl next door," and the "good mother." If these constructions of reality are opposed, they both depict "a confident woman" having relatively more breastfeeding experience than most of Quebec women. Finally, the development of the 2012 campaign raises some issues about the promotion of breastfeeding: preferred choice of a commercial approach to promote breastfeeding, economics issues, the consequences of public health campaign, as well as their effectiveness.

References

Agence de la santé et des services sociaux de Montréal. (2012). *Moi aussi j'allaite… Allaiter, c'est glamour,* Direction de la santé publique de Montréal. Retrieved from http://www.youtube.com/watch?v=WpivMPwMOGw

Agence de la santé et des services sociaux de Montréal. (2013). *Moi aussi j'allaite … Allaiter, parlons-en!,* Direction de la santé publique de Montréal. Retrieved from http://www.moiaussijallaite.com

Jodelet, D.. (with Moscovici, S., Ed.) (2003a). Représentation sociale: Phénomènes, concept et théorie. In *Psychologiesociale,* (p. 361-384). Paris: PUF.

Jodelet, D. (2003b). Représentations sociales: Un domaine en expansion. In *Les représentations sociales,* p. 47-78. Paris: PUF.

Ministère de la santé et des services sociaux. (2001). *L'allaitement maternel au Québec. Lignes directrices.* Québec: Gouvernement du Québec.

Ministère de la santé et des services sociaux du Québec. (2008). *Politique de périnatalité 2008-2018. Un projet porteur de vie*. Québec: Gouvernement du Québec.

Ministère de la santé et des services sociaux. (1997). *Priorités nationales de santé publique* 1997-2002. Québec: Gouvernement du Québec.

Ministère de la santé et des services sociaux du Québec. (2003). *Programme national de santé publique 2003-2012*. Québec: Gouvernement du Québec.

Ministère de la santé et des services sociaux du Québec. (2010). *Stratégies de mise en œuvre 2009-2012 de la Politique de périnatalité 2008-2018*. Québec: Gouvernement du Québec.

Statistiques Canada. (2013). *Tendances de l'allaitement maternel*. Retrieved from http://www.statcan.gc.ca/pub/82-624-x/2013001/article/11879-fra.pdf

The "Boob-Swinging Derelicts." Women's Lifestyle Blogs and the Ideology of Breastfeeding

Emily B. Anzicek

According to Internet data analytic firm comScore, North American women spent an average of 37.6 hours per month using the Internet in 2010. During those hours, 33.6% of women visited a "lifestyle" website (Abraham, Mörn, & Vollman, 2010). These websites are most often marketed to women and include coverage of a wide range of topics including fashion, celebrities, sex, parenting, etc. A subset of these lifestyle blogs is geared toward younger women, particularly those 18 to 35 years old. This study examines four of these lifestyle blogs that cater to younger women, *Jezebel*, *xoJane*, *The Hairpin*, and *The Gloss*, to explore what ideologies of breastfeeding are espoused by each.

Literature Review

The methodology of this study is situated in cultural studies. As such, I see cultural texts as value-laden, normalizing particular ideologies. In cultural studies, we see popular texts as important because they constitute so much of a person's everyday life. We can see Internet texts as perhaps even more dominant than others now, since the Internet is such an all-consuming form of media. In their discussion of the importance of the popular, Durham and Kellner argue that popular texts are prejudicial of difference (from the dominant), and have the power to influence how people think and act (Durham, & Kellner, 2001). In the scope of this study, I argue that currently, breast-feeding is not the ideologically dominant approach to infant feeding, so therefore, popular texts are prejudicial against breastfeeding. As such, breastfeeding rates in the United States could be affected by this prejudicial approach. Furthermore, Durham and Kellner argue that popular texts reinforce dominant ideologies, naturalizing dominant values (2001). In terms of breastfeeding, within popular texts, formula-feeding becomes the "natural" approach to infant feeding.

Social norms, or ideologies, are the biggest barriers to breast-feeding that American women experience. Breastfeeding activist group, Best for Babes, refers to these as "cultural booby traps," or cultural barriers to breastfeeding success ("What are the Booby Traps," n.d.). Some of the cultural barriers Best for Babes identifies include horror stories told by friends about breastfeeding, overzealous or "militant" breastfeeding advocates, and large amounts of misinformation online ("What are the Booby Traps," n.d.). *The Surgeon General's Call to Action to Support Breastfeeding* (U.S. Department of Health and Human Services, 2011) also identifies social norms and lack of social support as major barriers to breastfeeding success. Many scholars and activists have noted that breastfeeding is not perceived as normal,or typical, in the United States. As a result, women experience problems breastfeeding in public, expressing milk at work is frequently made difficult, and women are rarely allowed to bring babies to work to feed at the breast, and media images show babies drinking from bottles and breastfeeding as difficult.

Method

For the purposes of this study, I define women's lifestyle blogs as those marketed towards and framed for young women that focus on a wide range of information and topics, including sex, fashion, celebrity, and careers. I selected this wider range of topics because I am interested in how ideology affects women's perspectives on breastfeeding before they're pregnant or nursing because I believe that this affects breast-feeding success as well. Parenting websites or mommy blogs would likely not reach pre-parenting young women, and would therefore give more of a perspective on ideologies among mothers, not young women in general.

I selected *xoJane, The Hairpin, The Gloss, and Jezebel* because they are particularly popular with women 18 to 35 in the United States (as a matter of fact, Quantcast ranks Jezebel as the 139th most visited website in the U.S.). We can look at demographics for these via Quant-cast, a leading digital advertising company that specializes in audience measurement.

xoJane does not allow Quantcast to provide its numbers to the public, and they did not respond to my request to access their data. So their information comes from their ownership group, Say Media. Unfor-tunately, that means we can't get as specific with them. According to Say Media, *xoJane* averages 4 million monthly readers. As of March 2014, the website's Facebook page notes more than 42,000 "fans," and *xoJane's* Twitter lists more than 31,000 followers.

TheHairpin.com is owned by Federated Media Network, which also includes websites *The Awl* (general interest), *Splitsider* (humor), *The Billfold* (personal finance), and *Wirecutter* (tech). *The Hairpin* reaches 600,000 to 700,000 unique visitors (known in industry parlance as "uniques") monthly: 73% of the users are female, 47% are 18 to 34 years old (15% below 18, so 62% fall in that most likely pre-parent group), and 76% of their readers do not have children.

Jezebel.com is owned by Gawker Media, which also includes websites like *Gawker* (New York and Media gossip and info), *Deadspin* (sports and men's general interest), and *Gizmodo* (tech). *Jezebel* reaches about 12,500,000 uniques per month. Its readers are 66% female, 48% 18 to 34 years old (15% under 18), and 74% do not have children.

TheGloss.com is owned by Alloy Media, which also owns *Crushable* (entertainment), *Smosh* (comedy), and *The Escapist* (gaming). This website reaches about 1.3 million uniques per month. Its readers are 70% female, 46% 18-25 years old (15% below 18), and 72% have no children.

For the purposes of this study, I examined every article from these websites that featured breastfeeding as the main topic (not those that mentioned breastfeeding in passing, or did not report any in-depth information about the topic), dating back to 2011. I looked for major themes about breastfeeding, the type of language used to describe it, and how particular writers from each site framed breastfeeding.

Results and Discussion

The blogs analyzed for this study were largely unsupportive of and negative towards breastfeeding. Several themes emerged from this analysis. The first of these themes is that breastfeeding activists and supporters are the enemy. Labeled with such loaded terms as "Gestapo" (Morrissey, 2012, April), "lactivist cunts" (Morrissey, 2012, December), "dick-measurers" (Westervelt, 2013), and other rude terms, breastfeeding supporters and activists are situated as being against the breastfeeding mother, making her life more difficult, and making her feel guilty and inadequate, rather than helping her succeed. These supporters are accused of pressuring mothers and guilt-tripping them by throwing statistics and research, and by pointing out problems with formula.

Another theme is that breastfeeding itself is portrayed as negative, but not the cultural, social, and economic pressures that make breastfeeding difficult for American women. There is nothing wrong with a mother discussing her struggles and difficulties with breastfeeding. In fact, those kinds of stories can be empowering and beneficial to breast-feeding moms. The problem comes when the act of breastfeeding is framed as the problem (painful, inconvenient, hard, destructive to marriages, as in many articles across multiple of the analyzed blogs), instead of the "booby traps" that make it hard for women (for example, women aren't exposed to breastfeeding; the female body, and the breasts in particular, is highly sexualized; lack of paid maternity leave; lack of policies in the workplace that would allow women to feed their babies or express milk).

A final theme is that women who breastfeed will be socially ostra-cized, criticized, and seen as weird by the majority of the world around them. This theme is clearly illustrated by an *xoJane* article by Théri-ault, in which the author notes that, "People are fucking weird about breastfeeding" (2013). When so many articles portray breastfeeding women as non-normative and different, they are situated as the other. Seeing breastfeeding as not the norm can make it more difficult for young women to even consider breastfeeding. Breastfeeding past the age of 1 is portrayed as even more unusual, with multiple articles implying that people find "extended breastfeeding" to be "creepy," "weird," and "not normal" (Morrissey, 2013; Nelson, 2011; Peck, 2012; Thériault, 2013).

Conclusion

The blogs analyzed here are commercial, for-profit entities that rely on advertising and page views. Breastfeeding articles tend to be contro-versial in the current climate, and therefore, attract large numbers of page views, particularly when discourse becomes heated in the comments sections, which are very important and active parts of many of these sites. Breastfeeding activists, scholars, and supporters who use these websites can influence editors to accept more voices on breastfeeding, particularly more positive voices. *Jezebel,* in particular, has a very strong and thriving commenter community. While it is very difficult to get a pro-breastfeeding comment any attention due to their commenting format, enough positive comments can make a difference, and potentially elevate the discourse among users. Breastfeeding supporters who write about breastfeeding can submit work to these more mainstream sites in an attempt to get more positive and supportive voices heard on these issues, rather than simply contributing to sites that are already supportive. Social media (Twitter and Facebook especially) can be powerful tools to question and critique the arguments presented on lifestyle blogs. Supporters and activists should also seek to talk to young women about the information they're getting about breastfeeding, and how it affects them. With so many pre-parental users, these websites serve as a powerful source of information about motherhood and breastfeeding. We have to be aware of their ideologies, and how those may be impacting what their young female users believe to be true and normal about infant feeding.

References

Abraham, L. B., Mörn, M. P., & Vollman, A. (2010). *Women on the Web: How women are shaping the Internet*. Reston, VA: comScore.

Durham, M. G., & Kellner, D. (2001). Adventures in media and cultural studies: Introducing the key works. In M.G. Durham & D. Kellner (Eds.), *Media and cultural studies: Key works* (pp. 1-29). Malden, MA: Blackwell. Jezebel.com. (n.d.). Retrieved from https://www.quantcast.com/jezebel.com

Morrissey, T. E. (2012, April 11). *Breastfeeding Gestapo moves to ban free formula samples from hospitals*. Retrieved from http://jezebel.com/5900729/breastfeeding-gestapo-moves-to-ban-free-formula-samples-from-hospitals

Morrissey, T. E. (2012, December 17). *Fuck you, breastfeeding*. Retrieved from http://jezebel.com/5968243/fuck-you-breastfeeding

Morrissey, T. E. (2013, May 23). *Sorry lactation mafia: Neanderthals breastfed for only about a year*. Retrieved from http://jezebel.com/sorry-lactation-mafia-neanderthals-breastfed-for-only-509489312

Nelson, E. (2011, October 18). *It happened to me: I breast-fed my child until she was 4.* Retrieved from http://www.xojane.com/it-happened-to-me/it-happened-me-i-breast-fed-my-child-until-she-was-4

Peck, J. (2012, May 10). *America shows its weird relationship with boobs by "ew-ing"* Time *breastfeeding cover.* Retrieved from http://www.thegloss.com/2012/05/10/culture/time-breastfeeding-cover-reactions-822/ Thegloss.com. (n.d.). Retrieved from https://www.quantcast.com/thegloss.com

TheHairpin.com. (n.d.). Retrieved from https://www.quantcast.com/thehairpin.com

Thériault, A. (2013, February 25). *I am breastfeeding a two-year-old and it's not gross (I promise).* Retrieved from http://www.xojane.com/family/i-am-breastfeeding-a-two-year-old-and-its-not-gross-i-promise

U.S. Department of Health and Human Services. (2011). *The Surgeon General's Call to Action to Support Breastfeeding.* Washington, D.C.: U.S. Department of Health and Human Services, Office of the Surgeon General.

Westervelt, A. (2013, December 7). *Let's stop making breastfeeding the female version of dick measuring.* Retrieved from http://www.xojane.com/issues/lets-stop-making-breastfeeding-the-female-version-of-dick-measuring

What are the booby traps? (n.d.). Retrieved from http://www.bestforbabes.org/what-are-the-booby-traps/xoJane. (n.d.). About [Facebook page]. Retrieved from https://www.facebook.com/xoJanexoJane. (n.d.). Profile [Twitter page]. Retrieved from https://twitter.com/xojanedotcom

xoJane: The fastest growing women's lifestyle brand on the web. (n.d.). Retrieved from http://www.saymedia.com/xojane-0

Breastfeeding as Spectacle: How Media Depictions of Extreme Breastfeeding Discourage "Regular" Women

Katherine A. Foss

Forty-eight U.S. states have legislation that protects a woman's right to breastfeed in public (Li, Hsia, Fridinger, Benton-Davis, & Grummer-Strawn, 2004). Yet, despite this legal approval, nursing in public is still highly frowned upon. For example, a survey by Li and colleagues (2004) found only 43% of participants believed that mothers should be able to nurse in public. Furthermore, people are not even comfortable with mediated sightings of breastfeeding. In the survey by Li and colleagues, over 70% of respondents did not agree with the statement, "It is appropriate to show a woman breastfeeding her baby on TV programs" (Li et al., 2004). Unfortunately, this negativity has been translated to real-life interactions, in which women have been illegally ordered to either cover up, or vacate businesses, for breastfeeding (Harris, 2009; Harding, 2009; Maddux, 2009). Furthermore, the perception that breastfeeding is somehow obscene has left some women feeling vulnerable or uncomfortable nursing in public (Sheeshka et al., 2001).

This contradiction between the legal state of breastfeeding, and the lack of widespread cultural acceptance, has had dire consequences. Breastfeeding is considered such a vital part of health that the Surgeon General released a *Call to Action to Support Breastfeeding* in 2011. The American Academy of Pediatrics (AAP), among others, agree that breastfeeding rates are alarmingly low (American Academy of Pediatrics, 2005). Studies have shown that even people who are not in health care, and are not parents, understand that breastfeeding is beneficial (Kavanagh, Lou, Nicklas, Habibi, & Murphy, 2012; Marrone, Vogeltanz-Holm, & Holm, 2008; Spear, 2007). While most American women attempt to nurse, only 33% are exclusively breast-feeding at 3 months ("Breastfeeding Report Card," 2010). By 6 months, this number drops to only 13.3% (Centers for Disease Control and Prevention, 2010). Given that the extensive benefits of breastfeeding increase dramatically with duration, these low rates are now considered a public health issue.

Conflicting media messages help explain the negative cultural attitudes that hinder successful breastfeeding. The Surgeon General's report, as well as the AAP, have criticized the current news-and-entertainment media for negatively depicting breastfeeding, while presenting formula as the "normal" means of infant feeding (American Academy of Pediatrics, 2005; U.S. Department of Health and Human Services, 2011). Scholarly research on media's portrayals of breastfeeding supports the conclusion that the media have normalized formula, while blocking marketing campaigns that highlight the risk of not breastfeeding (Brown & Peuchaud, 2008; Foss, 2012; Foss, 2010; Wolf, 2007). Furthermore, media exaggerate "dangers" of breastfeeding (Hausman, 2003). When news-and-entertainment discourse tout "breast is best," it emphasizes breastfeeding's obstacles, while ignoring common solutions (Foss, 2013; Frerichs, Andsager, Campo, Aquilino, & Dyer, 2006; Potter, Sheeshka, & Valaitis, 2000; Young, 1990).

Media messages have also presented a narrow image of the "normalized breastfeeding mother." She is usually a married, professional, adult Caucasian, nursing her infant in the hospital (Foss,

2013). In recent years, this normalized nursing relationship has been reinforced by another type of mother—the spectacle—whose breast-feeding counters normative behavior to such an extreme that she is to be jeered at, and publicly ridiculed. This project analyzes the dichotomy of breastfeeding coverage in popular media, examining the media content, media coverage of the content, and readers' comments of three "spectacle" events, exploring how this media discourse polarizes women, and delegitimizes extended breastfeeding, hindering efforts to educate and support breastfeeding in American society.

In 2006, a British documentary, *Extraordinary Breastfeeding*, was released, covering the stories of women who nursed older children (Buchanan, 2006). An excerpt of this film, labeled "Breastfeeding at 8," was posted on Youtube, and has since received over 42.5 million views, and nearly 86,000 comments. On May 21, 2012, the cover of *Time* magazine featured a woman nursing a 3-year-old, with the title, "Are you Mom enough?" Backlash ensued, with individual readers and other media outlets extensively criticizing the photo. *YahooNews!*'s coverage of the story received more than 17,000 viewer comments, questioning the mother's psychological state, *Time* magazine's decision to print the photo, and the practice of extended breastfeeding overall. Similarly, in July 2012, an episode of the reality program, *Strange Sex,* also featured "extreme breastfeeding," showcasing a man who drinks human milk, sparking online debate about the function and sexuality of breastfeeding. As with the other two events, viewers of the online stories in the *Huffington Post,* and of the Youtube clip, left numerous comments on the "erotic breastfeeding" in the show.

The documentary, *Time* cover, and reality show present breast-feeding as deviant within the original content. For example, the Youtube description under "Breastfeeding at 8" is "Kids who are a little too attached." Likewise, the *Time* cover features the head-line, "Are you Mom Enough?" next to the image of an older child breastfeeding, conveying that the behavior does not conform to conventional expectations. The inclusion of "erotic breastfeeding" in a show entitled *Strange Sex* marks it as deviant as well.

Newspapers, blogs, and online communities have criticized these breastfeeding women in outlets ranging from *Forbes* magazine to parenting blogs. Writers distinguish between appropriate ages for breastfeeding, and what they consider to be "too old." The headline of *The Telegraph* article about Veronica Robinson (from "Breastfeeding at 8") states, "There comes a point when breast is not best" (Palmer, 2006). In the body of the article, writer Alison Palmer directly criticizes Robinson's choice with "I love to see a woman breastfeeding her baby whenever and wherever, just as God intended. But the operative word is 'baby.' Surely I'm not wrong to feel slightly repulsed by a woman being suckled by a child who can walk, talk and, in some cases, tie her own shoelaces?" She follows her remarks with a quote from a parenting psychologist who agrees with her repulsion.

Most of the reader comments of the "Breastfeeding at 8," and the *Time* magazine article also ridicule the children's ages. Viewers made 85, 972 comments about the Youtube video, most of which were negative. For example: "This is not normal," "Even without someone telling me this is wrong, when I see something like it, it gives me a weird, creepy feeling, and that's how I know it's not normal," and "This is gross." Similar comments were made for the *Time* cover—its *Huffington Post* story resulted in more than 4,000 messages, again, mostly negative, with statements such as, "When you look at best practices, sticking your boob in a preschool age child is not developmentally appropriate—EVER!" and "Breastfeeding until 5-years-old is NOT normal. Kids must be weaned at a reasonable age, 2 at the latest." While some readers wrote in favor of extended breastfeeding, they were quickly bombarded with negative feedback. For example, one reader remarked, "People are so upset over this, but will drink hormone and drug laden milk from another species, get a clue people, your worldview is upside down!" Another reader responded, "Yeah, call me silly and strange, but I don't want to drink my mother's breastmilk," ending the conversation.

Many of the media messages even imply sexual perversion for the breastfeeding women. *FoxNews* writer Keith Ablow argued, "The truth is that what *Time* magazine may have unwittingly captured, and been party to, was a grotesque form of psychological abuse" (2012). Reader feedback suggested similar responses. One person wrote (about Veronica Robinson) "She should be arrested for sexual abuse." Others remarked at how the breastfeeding mothers continue for their pleasure, not their babies, ignoring the numerous emotional and health benefits of extended breastfeeding.

Yet for the "erotic breastfeeding" on *Strange Sex*, media coverage and readers were surprisingly indifferent to a man "treating" his erectile dysfunction by drinking his wife's human milk. Despite the program title *Strange Sex*, most media outlets either ignored the show, or appeared neutral on the topic. For example, *Huffington Post* used the title "Breastfeeding Man: Jeff says drinking wife Michelle's human milk helped his erectile dysfunction" (Hanson, 2012). Many of the 395 comments suggested that Jeff's behavior was "normal," with remarks like, "Sucking on a woman's breasts gives a man an erection?! I had no idea!" and "Wow. Boobs in my face would cure ED for me too. LOL." Another reader wrote, "Just when I think I've heard it all. I guess as long as no one is hurt, and both are willing, whatever floats their boat." Other readers agreed, applauding them for identifying a fetish that worked for them.

Overall, the Youtube video, the *Time* magazine cover, and the *Strange Sex* "erotic breastfeeding" all marked certain breastfeeding relationships as "deviant"—nursing into the preschool years or breast-feeding a spouse. Yet the media coverage and reading responses were noticeably different, depending on who was breastfed. People were appalled by the nursing children, as stories of these cases exploded online, and readers rushed to leave their negative remarks. At the same time, the "breastfeeding man," who previously drank his wife's blood (which is usually considered taboo), received very little criticism, reinforcing breastfeeding as a sexual act, possibly more accepted as a tool for adult pleasure than children's nourishment.

Drawing from previous studies on media's depictions of breast-feeding, we then have a clear dichotomy of messages—the normalized nursing newborn, and at the other end of the spectrum, the "deviant" extended breastfeeding older child, with few messages in-between. With mainstream media messages rarely representing experiences between the newborn nursling and the "extreme" cases, breastfeeding is presented as an either/or choice, polarizing the extremists from tentative new mothers. The lack of a range of breastfeeding experiences, paired with the demonization of extended breastfeeding, likely explains why so many people are uncomfortable with breastfeeding, despite the laws that protect it.

References

Ablow, K. (2012, May 11). Forget the breast, what about the boy? *FoxNews*. Retrieved from http://www.foxnews.com/opinion/2012/05/11/time-magazine-cover-forget-breast-what-about-boy/

American Academy of Pediatrics. (2005). Breastfeeding and the use of human milk. *Pediatrics, 115*, 496–506.

Centers for Disease Control and Prevention. (2010). Breastfeeding Report Card. United States. Retrieved from http://www.cdc.gov/breastfeeding/pdf/BreastfeedingReportCard2010.pdf

Brown, J., & Peuchaud, S. (2008). Media and breastfeeding: Friend or foe? *International Journal of Breastfeeding, 3*(15). Retrieved from: http://internationalbreastfeedingjournal.com/content/3/1/15

Buchanan, K. (2006). *Extraordinary breastfeeding* [film]. RDF Media: Blackburn, Lancashire, England.

Foss, K. A. (2013). "That's not a beer bong, it's a breast pump!" Representations of breastfeeding in prime-time fictional television. *Health communication, 28*(4), 329-340.

Foss, K. (2012). Breastfeeding in the Baby Block: Using reality television to effectively promote breastfeeding, Chapter 20. In P.H. Smith, B.L. Hausman & M. Labbok (Eds.), *Beyond health, beyond choice: Breastfeeding constraints and realities.* Rutgers University Press.

Foss, K. (2010). Perpetuating scientific motherhood: Infant feeding discourse in *Parents* Magazine, 1930-2007. *Women & Health, 50*(3), 297-311.

Frerichs, L., Andsager, J. L., Campo, S., Aquilino, M., & Dyer, C. S. (2006). **Framing breastfeeding and formula-feeding messages in popular U.S. magazines.** *Women & Health, 44*(1), 95-118.

Hanson, H. (2012, July 12). Breastfeeding man: Jeff says drinking wife Michelle's milk helped his erectile dysfunction symptoms. *Huffington Post.* Retrieved from http://www.huffingtonpost.com/2012/07/11/breastfeeding-sex-erectile-dysfunction-jeff-michelle_n_1666073.html

Harding, K. (2009, December 7). Target calls cops on nursing mothers. *Broadsheet.* Retrieved from http://www.salon.com/life/broadsheet/feature/2009/12/07/target_breastfeeding/index.html

Harris, S. (2009, August 14). Breastfeeding battle at Chick-fil-A. *My Fox Orlando.* Retrieved from http://www.myfoxorlando.com/dpp/news/orange_news/081309_breastfeeding

Hausman, B. (2003). *Mother's milk: Breastfeeding controversies in American culture.* New York: Routledge.

Kavanagh, K. F., Lou, Z., Nicklas, J. C., Habibi, M. F., & Murphy, L. T. (2012). Breastfeeding knowledge, attitudes, prior exposure, and intent among undergraduate students. *Journal of Human Lactation, 28*(4), 556-564.

Li, R., Hsia, J., Fridinger, F., Benton-Davis, S., & Grummer-Strawn, L. (2004). Public beliefs about breastfeeding policies in various settings. *Journal of the American Dietetic Association, 104, 1162-1168.*

Maddux, S. (2009, August 19). Woman ousted from restaurant for breastfeeding. *NWI.com.* Retrieved from http://www.nwitimes.com/news/local/porter/article_515d04e0-58c5-5c13-b6fb-5c2d316c2d61.html

Marrone, S., Vogeltanz-Holm, N., & Holm, J. (2008). Attitudes, knowledge, and intentions related to breastfeeding among university undergraduate women and men. *Journal of human lactation, 24*(2), 186-192.

Palmer, A. (2006, February 3). There comes a point when breast is not best. *The Telegraph*. Retrieved from http://www.telegraph.co.uk/ health/3336122/There-comes-a-point-when-breast-is-not-best.html

Potter, B., Sheeshka, J., & Valaitis, R. (2000). Content analysis of infant feeding messages in a Canadian women's magazine, 1945 to 1995. *Journal of Nutrition Education, 32*, 196-203.

Sheeshka, J., Potter, B., Norrie, E., Valaitis, R., Adams, G., & Kuczynski, L. (2001). Women's experiences breastfeeding in public places. *Journal of Human Lactation, 17*, 31-38.

Spear, H. J. (2007). College students' experiences and attitudes regarding middle and high school–based breastfeeding education. *The Journal of School Nursing, 23*(5), 276-282.

U.S. Department of Health and Human Services. (2011). *The Surgeon General's Call to Action to Support Breastfeeding*. Washington, DC: U.S. Department of Health and Human Services, Office of the Surgeon General.

Wolf, J. B. (2007). Is breast really best? Risk and total motherhood in the national breastfeeding awareness campaign. *Journal of Health Politics, Policy, and Law, 32*(4), 595-636.

Young, K. (1990). American conceptions of infant development from 1955 to 1984: What the experts are telling parents. *Child Development, 61*, 17-28.

"F*** You, Breastfeeding": Anti-Breastfeeding Narratives in Online Feminist News Media

Spring-Serenity Duvall

Theoretical Foundations

In recent years, breastfeeding has gained widespread media prominence, creating controversies that elicit responses from feminist bloggers, journalists, pundits, celebrities, and activists. My project engages with feminist communications theory to critically analyze breastfeeding discourses that emerge in contemporary digital media outlets, such as *Jezebel* and *Feministing,* which self-identify as feminist productions. Despite NOW's official stance being pro-breastfeeding, and supportive of institutional reforms to facilitate breastfeeding flexibility, feminist bloggers and media outlets often disparage pro-breastfeeding policies, and promote an anti-breastfeeding perspective, continuing (to paraphrase Hausman, 2004) the public feminist bashing of maternalist practices. The tensions within contemporary conceptions of gender equality and feminism seem to suggest a post-feminist, and third-wave feminist belief that female empowerment is contingent upon liberation from childbearing, nurturing, and breastfeeding (Wolf, 2006).

The tensions between institutional directives that women should breastfeed and the economic, personal, and medical barriers that women face as they navigate whether to breastfeed, and for how long, contributes to the ongoing cultural dialogue about breastfeeding that suggests women are defined by their maternity. Maternal women are subjugated by the laws, policies, and culture that value her primarily as a vessel for gestating, birthing, and nurturing offspring. As both a biological function, and a socially constructed practice, "breastfeeding provides a focus that encourages us to see women's bodies at the center of the dilemmas of modern societies" (Hausman, 2004). Media stereotype, marginalize, sexualize, and demonize breastfeeding. This study employs a textual analysis of dominant themes across online feminist media outlets. Any effort to prescribe breastfeeding is met with ire, while women who have already chosen to breastfeed are supported.

Dominant Themes

Initial analysis shows that the narratives emerging from feminist media discourses about breastfeeding often perpetuate stereotypes of women being pitted against each other in a skirmish over individual choice, damaging the potential for societal-level interventions that might, as Wolf argues, "reopen a national dialogue about an array of currently dormant feminist goals" concerning workplace equality and women's health (2006, p. 416). There are three dominant themes in the pieces about breastfeeding that appear in *Jezebel* and *Feministing*, each converging to create an overall narrative that breastfeeding is a negative experience for women.

First, the continued taboo against breastfeeding is reflected in routine instances of women being forced to stop breastfeeding in public places, such as courthouses, department stores, and parks, where they have every legal right to breastfeed. Reports in *Jezebel* and on *Feministing* defend these women's rights to breastfeed in any location without being harassed. Confining breastfeeding to lactation rooms, and "breastfeeding-friendly" spaces, can be problematic because it re-inscribes the bourgeois notions that ignore entire cultures of women around the world who breastfeed in crowded, noisy spaces. As Rose (2012) posits, "we must question whose interests are being served with distinctions of public/private and, moreover, what are the imbedded meanings of the reserving private space for lactating women?" (p. 51). By reporting on instances of women being told to cover up, stop nursing, or being shamed for nursing in public spaces, *Jezebel* and *Feministing* seem to promote the normalization of breastfeeding. Yet the emphasis on breastfeeding in public as a struggle in which women do experience shame, and are forced to defend themselves after or during the encounters, re-inscribes the perception that breastfeeding will be a contentious, negative experience for mothers. Women who breastfeed in public often experience feelings of shame, as they internalize cultural norms about "proper" (i.e., private) breastfeeding (Taylor & Wallace, 2012). By granting visibility primarily to negative breastfeeding experiences, these two online feminist news outlets perpetuate a narrative that breastfeeding in public will be a negative experience for mothers.

Second, personal narratives, written by senior staff at *Jezebel* and *Feministing,* focus on their own breastfeeding experiences as painful and difficult. These personal narratives occupy a more privileged position on the websites than the items that defend women's rights to breastfeed in public. Because the personal narratives are longer, more in-depth, and produced by senior staff, these items represent the authoritative voice of the websites themselves. By recounting their own painful, or disappointing physical and emotional struggles with breastfeeding, these writers create the narrative that even though they believe that other women have the right to breastfeed, they do not experience breastfeeding in a positive way themselves. Furthermore, their negative personal trials with breastfeeding have been exacerbated by feeling attacked and judged by pro-breastfeeding women or groups, who have treated them with condescension or pressure to breastfeed, even when they are physically incapable of doing so. Thus, accounts of negative experiences with breastfeeding also become infused with anger towards pro-breastfeeding messages.

Anger towards both the act of breastfeeding and breastfeeding advocates is expressed in aggressively sexualized language that may undermine claims throughout news reports, and personal narratives, that breastfeeding should be normalized and desexualized. The possible outcome is that, as with the first theme, the overall message sent to audiences is one in which a woman's experience with breast-feeding is difficult in its one right, and made worse by encounters with hurtful pro-breastfeeding messages.

Finally, commentary on both websites about pro-breastfeeding campaigns, and scientific inquiries about breastfeeding, engage in selective outrage that casts institutions as anti-woman. Authors lash out against policies, such as New York's breastfeeding promotion campaign, claiming that women are being "forced" to breastfeed as a form of gender oppression. Scientific findings regarding the limitations of breastfeeding, and evidence that supports the merits of formula-feeding, are reported gleefully as proof that pro-breastfeeding activists are wrong to advocate breastfeeding as the ideal form of infant feeding.

Implications

The tensions within feminisms about motherhood, and the stereo-types that dominate media messages about breastfeeding, may contribute to women internalizing judgments about the expectations of how feminists should perform motherhood. Survey results show that feminist mothers endorse attachment-parenting practices, such as breastfeeding, more than non-feminist mothers, yet also stereo-type "feminist mothers" as being anti-attachment parenting (Liss & Erchull, 2012). Thus, women who self-identify as feminist also choose attachment parenting approaches, yet believe that they may somehow be betraying feminist ideals by doing so, and may believe that other feminists would not support their mothering practices. It is possible that even feminist mothers think that there is a disconnect between their "feminist" (i.e., powerful, independent) selves, and their "mother" selves. The backlash from women and feminist groups also shows tensions within contemporary conceptions of gender equality and feminism that seem to suggest female empowerment is contingent upon liberation from childbearing, nurturing, and breastfeeding (Wolf, 2006). The dominant narrative that emerges in *Jezebel* and *Feministing* is one in which women were pitted against each other in a skirmish over individual choice, damaging the potential for societal level interventions that might, as Wolf argues "reopen a national dialogue about an array of currently dormant feminist goals" concerning workplace equality and women's health (2006, p. 416).

The complexities of negotiating dueling discourses that suggest that contemporary empowerment is dependent on either freedom from breastfeeding or freedom to breastfeed. It is particularly important to investigate the discourses about breastfeeding that dominate feminist media outlets because that content can potentially define feminist politics of breastfeeding in policy negotiations and popular imaginations. Furthermore, such media content can influence audiences and policy-makers who conflate an anti-breastfeeding perspective with feminist empowerment.

References

Hausman, B. L. (2004). The feminist politics of breastfeeding. *Australian Feminist Studies, 19*(45), 273-285.

Liss, M., & Erchull, M. J. (2012). Feminism and attachment parenting: Attitudes, stereotypes, and Misperceptions. *Sex Roles, 67*(3-4), 131-142.

Rose, L. M. (2012). Legally public but privately practiced: Segregating the lactating body. *Health Communication, 27*, 49-57.

Taylor, E. N., & Wallace, L. E. (2012). For shame: Feminism, breastfeeding advocacy, and maternal guilt. *Hypatia, 27*(1), 76-98.

Wolf, J. (2006). What feminists can do for breastfeeding and what breastfeeding can do for feminists. *Signs: Journal of Women in Culture and Society, 31*(2), 397-424.

Concluding Comments

This volume only begins to explore the possible areas of partnership with other sectors and disciplines. We know that breastfeeding has a profound contribution for maternal and child health, and yet it is a biological issue unique to the female. Where does it truly fit into our societies, with emerging markets and economic underpinnings? Perhaps when there is a price tag associated with the productive reality of the contribution to society that is offered by reproduction, child development, health, and survival, and maternal-health cost savings associated with breastfeeding, then our societies will provide all women with support for the normalcy and importance of healthy replacement fertility.

The Breastfeeding and Feminism International Conference seeks to advance social, health, and feminist aspects of breastfeeding in order to achieve an optimal breastfeeding norm. We have approached this issue from several "frames," from feminist empowerment, to health care, per se, to sociological examination, to global rapprochement, and yet, much remains to be done to create a commonality of purpose.

This volume is the fifth publication of edited proceedings from the Breastfeeding and Feminism International Conference (BFIC). [1] We hope that you found the selected papers of interest. For further readings on these and related topics, you may wish to seek out and explore the series of publications that emerged from these conferences, and that you will join us at future Breastfeeding and Feminism International Conferences, and/or visit the conference website[2] or Facebook page[3].

Miriam Labbok, MD, MPH, IBCLC   Paige Hall Smith, PhD

---

1   Previous conference outcomes were presented as 1) a series of papers based on the 3rd conference (2007) that aimed to reposition breastfeeding as a valued part of women's (re)productive lives and rights, published in the *International Breastfeeding Journal*, starting with: Labbok, M.H., Smith, P.H., & Taylor, E.C. (2008). Breastfeeding and feminism: A focus on reproductive health, rights and justice. *International Breastfeeding Journal*,3:8, doi:10.1186/1746-4358-3-8, 2)

The 5th conference resulted in an edited book: Smith, P.H., Hausman, B.L., & Labbok, M.H. (Eds). (2012). *Beyond health, beyond choice:Breastfeeding constraints and realities,* New Brunswick, NJ: Rutgers University Press.

The 7th conference resulted in a presentation at U.S. Breastfeeding Committee and a paper entitled, "Considering Women in Advancing the *Surgeon General's Call to Action,*" addressing women's reactions to the 20 action areas.

The 8th conference resulted in another edited book. Smith, P.H., & Labbok, M.H. (Eds.) 2015, *It takes a Village The role of the greater community in inspiring and empowering women to breastfeed.* Amarillo TX: Praeclarus Press.

And the 9th conference resulted in the present volume.
2   http://breastfeedingandfeminism.org/
3   https://www.facebook.com/BreastfeedingAndFeminismInternationalConference

www.ingramcontent.com/pod-product-compliance
Lightning Source LLC
Chambersburg PA
CBHW071636270326
41928CB00010B/1943